Adequate HLA Matching in Keratoplasty

Developments in Ophthalmology

Vol. 36

Series Editor   *W. Behrens-Baumann*, Magdeburg

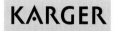

KARGER

Basel · Freiburg · Paris · London · New York ·
New Delhi · Bangkok · Singapore · Tokyo · Sydney

Adequate HLA Matching in Keratoplasty

Volume Editor   *R. Sundmacher*, Düsseldorf

17 figures and 11 tables, 2003

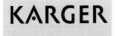

Basel · Freiburg · Paris · London · New York ·
New Delhi · Bangkok · Singapore · Tokyo · Sydney

··················

Prof. Dr. R. Sundmacher

Universität Düsseldorf
Klinik für Augenheilkunde
Moorenstrasse 5
D–40225 Düsseldorf

Continuation of 'Bibliotheca Ophthalmologica', 'Advances in Ophthalmology', and
'Modern Problems in Ophthalmology'

Founded 1926 as 'Abhandlungen aus der Augenheilkunde und ihren Grenzgebieten' by
C. Behr, Hamburg and *J. Meller*, Wien

Former Editors: *A. Brückner*, Basel (1938–1959); *H.J.M. Wewe*, Utrecht (1938–1962);
H.M. Dekking, Groningen (1954–1966); *E.B. Streiff*, Lausanne (1954–1979);
J. François, Gand (1959–1979); *J. van Doaesschate*, Utrecht (1967–1971);
M.J. Roper-Hall, Birmingham (1966–1980); *H. Sautter*, Hamburg (1966–1980);
W. Straub, Marburg a.d. Lahn (1981–1993)

Library of Congress Cataloging-in-Publication Data

Adequate HLA matching in keratoplasty / volume editor, R. Sundmacher.
    p. ; cm. – (Developments in ophthalmology, ISSN 0250–3751 ; v. 36)
 Includes bibliographical references and index.
 ISBN 3805574878 (hard cover : alk. paper)
   1. Cornea–Transplantation–Immunological aspects. 2. HLA histocompatibility
antigens. I. Sundmacher, Rainer, 1943– II. Series.
   [DNLM: 1. Corneal Transplantation–immunology. 2. Histocompatibility Testing. 3.
HLA Antigens. WW 220 A232 2003]
 RE336 .A33 2003
 617.7′190592–dc21
                                                                    2002034061

    Bibliographic Indices. This publication is listed in bibliographic services, including Current Contents® and Index Medicus.

    Drug Dosage. The authors and the publisher have exerted every effort to ensure that drug selection and dosage set forth in this text are in accord with current recommendations and practice at the time of publication. However, in view of ongoing research, changes in government regulations, and the constant flow of information relating to drug therapy and drug reactions, the reader is urged to check the package insert for each drug for any change in indications and dosage and for added warnings and precautions. This is particularly important when the recommended agent is a new and/or infrequently employed drug.

    © Copyright 2003 by S. Karger AG, P.O. Box, CH–4009 Basel (Switzerland)
www.karger.com
Printed in Switzerland on acid-free paper by Reinhardt Druck, Basel
ISSN 0250–3751
ISBN 3–8055–7487–8

Contents

Preface

The practical value of using HLA-matched grafts for corneal transplantation has been a matter of controversy from the beginning and the vast majority of corneal surgeons and directors of cornea banks still seem to believe that no proof exists that HLA matching may contribute significantly to transplant survival. Whereas in most clinical fields we can nowadays state that medical progress follows universal mainstream lines, this does not seem to be the case with HLA matching and corneal transplantation. A growing Central European group has worked out ways and rules how to achieve a significant contribution to long-term corneal transplant survival by HLA matching, while in other parts of the world, and also in the USA, these results seem to have been partly ignored or misjudged. On the occasion of the Meeting of the German Ophthalmological Society held in Berlin in September 2001, a group of 'HLA promoters' gathered to present and discuss their latest results. One of the main problems in understanding past developments in HLA lies in the fact that the literature is too diffuse, and therefore the information available to individual researchers is often inadequate. We thought it desirable to offer a compilation of some of the important aspects in this volume, to increase understanding and promote discussion. We hope this book will contribute to this aim, and extend the perception of HLA matching as a positive contributory factor in corneal transplants, provided it is properly understood and employed.

Rainer Sundmacher, Düsseldorf

Sundmacher R (ed): Adequate HLA Matching in Keratoplasty.
Dev Ophthalmol. Basel, Karger, 2003, vol 36, pp 1–4

....

Introduction

Rainer Sundmacher, Thomas Reinhard

Eye Hospital and Lions Cornea Bank North Rhine-Westphalia,
Heinrich Heine University, Düsseldorf, Germany

Almost one century after the first successful penetrating keratoplasty [1], immune reactions are still a major problem in normal-risk as well as in high-risk situations [2–4]. Due to the immune privilege of the cornea and the anterior chamber [5–8], topical corticosteroid prophylaxis over some months post-operatively has been supposed to sufficiently limit this complication [9, 10]. On an average, however, in normal-risk keratoplasty about 18% and in high-risk situations up to 75% of the patients still experience immune reactions, often with subsequent graft failure [2–4].

In order to further reduce the immunologic threat effectively, topical and/or systemic immunosuppressives may be intensified and administered in a more prolonged way. This, however, will often go along with a markedly enhanced risk of severe side effects. The only alternative or adjunct to this drug-intensifying strategy, which has become increasingly successful and thus popular during the last decades, would be a more efficient use of the still mostly unexploited potentials of HLA matching.

The basically beneficial effect of HLA class I and II matching in renal transplantation has been undisputed [11]. Numerous penetrating keratoplasty studies performed within the past three decades, however, gave contradictory results as to the usefulness of HLA matching in corneal grafting [12–25]. This calls for explanation, which may be threefold:

(1) In multicenter studies with up to 200 centers and up to 400 surgeons, different surgical experience and techniques may influence the outcome [26].

(2) Most studies were performed in high-risk patients who do not only have an elevated risk of immune reactions but also – and often at a higher degree – additional non-immunologic risk factors such as surface disorders (e.g. in atopic keratoconjunctivitis or in limbal stem cell deficiencies), glaucoma problems or viral or microbial recurrences [27]. HLA matching has,

of course, no influence whatsoever on these additional non-immunological risk factors, which by themselves often lead to irreversible graft failure. In cases with most severe lime burns, e.g., the risk of non-immunologic graft failure from limbal stem cell deficiency alone will approach 100% without any necessity of additional damage by immune reactions. If, therefore, only the total of graft failures is registered this total will give no really reliable information on the percentage of underlying immunological causes. And even if it was tried to differentiate between immunological and non-immunological causes of graft failures, then such attempts must have remained mostly insufficient as it is evident that many authors have not even known important non-immunological causes for graft failure, e.g. the very high risk of non-immunological graft failure from undetected, untreated secondary glaucoma.

(3) Finally, the quality of HLA typing in many previous studies has been a matter of prime concern. In some studies, HLA typing was performed in laboratories which were not quality controlled. As far as the reliance of the CCTS data is concerned, concordance between the published original data and control data gained by retyping with modern techniques later on was only 55% [28, 29]. Völker-Dieben et al. [29] have demonstrated that faulty HLA-DR typing in only 5% of the cases suffices to abrogate the beneficial effect of HLA-DR matching. HLA typing on a molecular genetic basis is nowadays regarded to be the safest way to avoid typing errors in HLA class II. This is especially true when blood obtained up to 72 h after the donor's death is analyzed [11, 30]. In previous keratoplasty studies, however, HLA typing had been performed almost exclusively serologically.

In this book, Ilias Doxiadis (Leiden, The Netherlands) will present modern and reliable HLA-typing techniques as the basis for optimal HLA matching. On this basis the effectiveness of HLA matching in high- and normal-risk keratoplasty patients will be shown in three monocenter studies with more than 2,000 patients by Houdijn Beekhuis (Rotterdam, The Netherlands), Hennie Völker-Dieben (Amsterdam, The Netherlands) and Thomas Reinhard (Düsseldorf, Germany). The decision whether or not a patient should wait for an HLA-matched corneal graft will not only depend on the calculable immunological risks but also – and often even more decisively – on logistic availability aspects. Daniel Böhringer (Düsseldorf, Germany) will demonstrate a calculation method for the waiting time for an HLA-matched corneal graft for every individual patient so that the patient may discuss and decide with his ophthalmologist whether he should plan for a matched graft or rather prefer a random graft and rely on the potentials of modern medical immune therapy alone. According to Theo de By (Leiden, The Netherlands) recent doubling of HLA-typed corneal grafts allocated by Bio Implant Services (Leiden, The Netherlands) has already allowed to considerably reduce the waiting time for patients scheduled for matching. Frans Claas (Leiden, The Netherlands) will present his fascinating concept of 'permissible' and 'taboo' HLA mismatches and its influence on future HLA-matching strategies. Wayne Streilein (Boston, Mass., USA) will show that beside major antigen matching, minor antigen matching may become interesting for penetrating keratoplasty patients in the future. And finally, Rainer Sundmacher (Düsseldorf, Germany) will sum up what he believes that the practical consequences should be of the above-presented results.

References

1 Zirm E: Eine erfolgreiche totale Keratoplastik. Graefes Arch Clin Exp Ophthalmol 1906;64: 581–593.
2 Hill JC: The use of cyclosporine in high-risk keratoplasty. Am J Ophthalmol 1989;107:506–510.
3 Hill JC: Systemic cyclosporine in high-risk keratoplasty. Short- versus long-term therapy. Ophthalmology 1994;101:128–133.
4 Reinhard T, Hutmacher M, Sundmacher R, Godehardt E: Akute und chronische Immunreaktionen nach perforierender Keratoplastik mit normalem Immunrisiko. Klin Monatsbl Augenheilkd 1997; 210:139–143.
5 Streilein J: Unraveling immune privilege. Science 1995;270:1158–1159.
6 Niederkorn JY, Mellon J: Anterior chamber-associated immune deviation promotes corneal allograft survival. Invest Ophthalmol Vis Sci 1996;36:1530–1540.
7 Yamada J, Streilein JW: Induction of anterior chamber-associated immune deviation by corneal allografts placed in the anterior chamber. Invest Ophthalmol Vis Sci 1997;38:2833–2843.
8 Sano Y, Okamoto S, Streilein JW: Induction of donor-specific ACAID can prolong orthotopic corneal allograft survival in 'high-risk' eyes. Curr Eye Res 1997;16:1171–1174.
9 Sundmacher R: Immunreaktionen nach Keratoplastik. Klin Monatsbl Augenheilkd 1977; 171:705–722.
10 Sundmacher R, Stefansson A, Mackensen G: Verlaufsbeobachtungen nach Keratoplastik. Fortschr Ophthalmol 1983;80:224–227.
11 Opelz G, Mytilineos J, Scherer S, Dunckley H, Trejaut J, Chapman J, Fischer G, Fae I, Middleton D, Savage D, Bignon JD, Bensa JC, Noreen H, Albert E, Albrecht G, Schwarz V: Analysis of HLA-DR matching in DNA-typed cadaver kidney transplants. Transplantation 1993;55:782–785.
12 Gibbs DC, Batchelor R, Werb A, Schlesinger W, Casey TA: The influence of tissue-type compatibility on the fate of full-thickness corneal grafts. Trans Ophthalmol Soc 1974;94:101–126.
13 Vannas S: Histocompatibility in corneal grafting. Invest Ophthalmol 1975;14:883–886.
14 Stark WJ, Hugh RT, Bias WB, Maumenee AE: Histocompatibility (HLA) antigens and keratoplasty. Am J Ophthalmol 1978;86:595–604.
15 Ehlers N, Kissmeyer-Nielsen F: Corneal transplantation and HLA histocompatibility. Acta Ophthalmol 1979;57:738–741.
16 Foulks GN, Sanfilippo FP, Locasio JA, MacQueen JM, Dawson DV: Histocompatibility testing for keratoplasty in high-risk patients. Ophthalmology 1983;90:239–244.
17 Sanfilippo F, MacQueen JM, Vaughn WK, Foulks GN: Reduced graft rejection with good HLA-A and -B matching in high-risk corneal transplantation. N Engl J Med 1986;315:29–35.
18 Völker-Dieben HJ, D'Amaro J, Kruit PJ, Lange P: Interaction between prognostic factors for corneal allograft survival. Transplant Proc 1989;21:3135–3138.
19 Boisjoly HM, Roy R, Bernard PM, Dubé I, Laughrea PA, Bazin R: Association between corneal allograft reactions and HLA compatibility. Ophthalmology 1990;97:1689–1698.
20 Baggesen K, Ehlers N, Lamm LU: HLA-DR/RFLP compatible corneal grafts. Acta Ophthalmol 1991;69:229–233.

21 Beekhuis WH, van Rij G, Renardel de Lavalette JG, Rinkel-van Driel E, Persijn G, D'Amaro J: Corneal graft survival in HLA-A- and HLA-B-matched transplantations in high-risk cases with retrospective review of HLA-DR compatibility. Cornea 1991;10:9–12.

22 CCTS: Effectiveness of histocompatibility matching in high-risk corneal transplantation. Arch Ophthalmol 1992;110:1392–1403.

23 Vail A, Gore SM, Bradley BA, Easty DL, Rogers CA, Armitage WJ: Conclusions of the corneal transplant follow-up study. Br J Ophthalmol 1997;81:631–636.

24 Hoffmann F, Pahlitzsch T: Predisposing factors in corneal graft rejection. Cornea 1989;8: 215–219.

25 Hoffmann F, Tregel M, Noske W, Bünte S: HLA-B and -DR match reduces the allograft rejection after keratoplasty. Ger J Ophthalmol 1994;3:100–104.

26 Gore SM, Vail A, Bradley BA, Rogers CA, Easty DL, Armitage WJ: HLA-DR matching in corneal transplantation: Systematic review of published data. Transplantation 1995;110:1392.

27 Reinhard T, Sundmacher R, Heering P: Systemic ciclosporin A in high-risk keratoplasties. Graefes Arch Clin Exp Ophthalmol 1996;234(suppl 1):115–121.

28 Hopkins KA, Maguire MG, Fink NE, Bias WB: Reproducibility of HLA-A, -B, and -DR typing using peripheral blood samples: Results of retyping in the CCTS. Hum Immunol 1992;22:132.

29 Völker-Dieben HJ, Claas FHJ, Schreuder GMT, Schipper RF, Pels E, Persijn GG, Smits J, D'Amaro J: Beneficial effect of HLA-DR matching on the survival of corneal allografts. Transplantation 2000;70:640–648.

30 Wernet P, Kögler G, Enczmann J, Kuhröber A, Knipper A, Bonte W, Reinhard T, Sundmacher R: Rapid method for successful HLA class I and II typing from cadaveric blood for direct matching in cornea transplantation. Graefes Arch Clin Exp Ophthalmol 1998;236:507–512.

Thomas Reinhard, MD
Eye Hospital and Lions Cornea Bank North Rhine-Westphalia,
Heinrich Heine University, D–40225 Düsseldorf (Germany)
Tel. +49 211 8118795, Fax +49 211 8118796, E-Mail thomas.reinhard@uni-duesseldorf.de

Sundmacher R (ed): Adequate HLA Matching in Keratoplasty.
Dev Ophthalmol. Basel, Karger, 2003, vol 36, pp 5–11

....

The Short Story of HLA and Its Methods

Ilias I.N. Doxiadis, Frans H.J. Claas

Department of Immunohaematology and Blood Transfusion,
Leiden University Medical Center, Leiden, The Netherlands

Abstract

Background: During the past 40 years, typing for the human leukocyte antigens (HLA) was done using serological techniques. Several improvements were achieved as to the efficiency and reliability of these techniques. One of the major drawbacks of serology, however, is the need of viable cells. Especially blood cells drawn from deceased donors, as are the usual source for typing of corneal donors, may have a grossly impaired viability and a reduced expression of antigens on their cell surface. This makes serological typing difficult and liable to errors. In the mid-1980s, molecular typing was first introduced in many laboratories. This first period dealt with the so-called *restriction fragment length polymorphism method*, a tedious method not suited for prospective typing. Only with the introduction of the polymerase chain reaction was the suitability of molecular techniques with respect to perspective typing achieved.

Methods: International workshops and the effort of many laboratories led to a standardization of the methods. External proficiency testing exercises on transplantation relevant procedures in the laboratories affiliated to transplantation centers and the introduction of an accreditation system in the USA and in Europe increased significantly the reliability of all relevant immunogenetical testing.

Results: To date, patients and prospective organ and tissue donors are typed in addition to serology also with molecular methods. Using these techniques, the reliability and reproducibility of HLA typing have reached levels of more than 98%. Even 8-day-old peripheral blood samples can now be typed routinely with these methods, formerly impossible by serology.

Conclusion: The laboratories affiliated to the transplantation centers are ready for high reliability testing of all HLA markers required by the clinic according to the results of controlled clinical long-term follow-up studies.

Experimental transfer of tumors from one mouse strain to the other led to the discovery of the major histocompatibility complex (MHC) [1]. In humans, the products of the MHC named human leukocyte antigens (HLA) were first described by Dausset [2] in 1954. The antibody recognized an antigen named MAC, today known as HLA-A2. On April 11, 1958, Mrs. v.d.H.B., 26 years old, was delivered of premature twins. Due to hemorrhage, an emergency blood transfusion was given. Within 1 h a severe transfusion reaction manifested itself by collapse, hypotension, nausea, vomiting, and shaking chill. Investigation of the reaction did not show the presence of blood group incompatibility. On the other hand, the presence of strong agglutinins, which could agglutinate the leukocytes of the donor, was demonstrated. The patient did not have a transfusion history, but six previous pregnancies [3, 4]. This discovery made clear that antibodies against components of the MHC can be formed during pregnancy and are directed against the paternal HLA antigens.

The Antigens

Klein et al. [5] first divided the MHC antigens (molecules) into different classes according to their expression pattern and association to other molecules. The class I molecules, expressed on almost all nucleated body cells, are composed of a heavy chain, encoded in the MHC region on chromosome 6 p (petit) band 22, a light chain, β_2-microglobulin, and a peptide of about 9–11 amino acid length. These molecules are the counterparts of the T-cell receptor on $CD8^+$ T cells, usually called cytotoxic T cells. MHC class I molecules transport intracellular peptides to the cell surface. In case of a viral infection of the cell, viral peptides are also transported to the cell surface together with all the other intracellular self peptides. There, the viral peptides (non-self) can be recognized by the cytotoxic T cells, leading to the destruction of the infected cell. The class I molecules represent the antigens HLA-A, B and C. Class II molecules are expressed on some specific cells, e.g. monocytes, activated T cells (in humans), and B cells. Furthermore, Langerhans' and dendritic cells express abundantly class II molecules. One can state that only antigen-presenting cells can/do have class II molecules on their cell surface. These are the antigens HLA-DR, DQ and DP.

Besides the 'classical' class I antigens HLA-A, B and C, additional class I molecules can be found on specific cells, like trophoblasts. These 'non-classical' class I antigens (HLA-E, F and G), can be seen as counterparts of the natural killer cells [6]. The 'classical' class I molecules are the counterparts of T cells, as stated above, but act also as targets for the natural killer cell. Obviously, T-cell receptors recognize other regions on the class I molecules than the natural

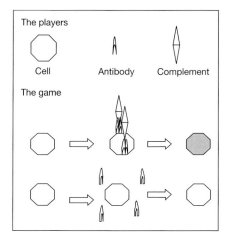

Fig. 1. The microdroplet assay or the game between cells, antibodies and complement. Complement can only be activated when antibodies have recognized their counterpart structures (antigen) on the cell surface. Perforine-like molecules make holes in the membrane through which a colored dye can enter.

killer cell. The best example represents the epitope Bw4, which cannot be recognized by the T cells but is one of the counterparts of the natural killer receptors.

Methods for Typing of HLA Antigens

Serologically Based Methods

HLA antigens were discovered by means of serological assays. At first the macro agglutination assay was used, for which large volumes of sera, 2 drops or about 100 µl and 2 drops of cells were used. In case of the presence of HLA antibodies, the cells agglutinated. It is obvious that not all antibodies could be detected by this method. Especially some antibodies of the IgG type might have escaped detection. Later, the method was miniaturized by Terasaki's group [7], who published in the early 1970s the currently used technique: the microdroplet assay, better known as the complement-dependent cytotoxicity assay (CDC). This assay is found in the literature and is also called the standard NIH (for National Institute of Health) technique or lymphocytotoxicity test (LCT). In short, sera (1 µl) are pre-dropped in special trays and the trays are stored frozen until use. In case of need, the trays are thawed and 1 µl of cells is added. After an incubation time of 30 min, 6 µl rabbit complement is given and the trays are further incubated at room temperature. Finally, a colored dye is added and the trays are ready for evaluation (schematically depicted in figure 1). This method is currently still used in the vast majority of HLA

AA pos.	77	80	81	82	83
B*3501	Ser	Asn	Leu	Arg	Gly
B*5301	Asn	Ile	Ala	Leu	Arg

Fig. 2. Serological difference between HLA-B35 and HLA-B53.

laboratories especially for typing of class I antigens and the cross-match prior to transplantation. For a comprehensive typing, sera from multiparous women, patients and monoclonal antibodies were screened against large panels of HLA-typed cells. Furthermore, the exchange of cells, reagents, and cells because of the International Histocompatibility Workshops [8], perhaps the best idea since the discovery of MHC, made HLA typing possible around the world.

Using serological methods, even very closely related antigens as shown in figure 2 could be identified. These antigens, HLA-B35 and HLA-B53, both closely related and according to their amino acid structure identical, differ in 5 amino acids in the region position 77–83, known as the Bw4/Bw6 epitopes, first described by van Rood in the example reported at the beginning of the present report. Following the nomenclature established during the International Histocompatibility Workshops, especially the HLA-A and HLA-B antigens were divided into the so-called 'broad' and splits. Every HLA 'broad' antigen, e.g. HLA-A9, was split into two or more other antigens, HLA-A23 and HLA-A24. This was made possible when additional sera were found and their reactivity established in one of the Workshops.

For typing of the class II antigens the isolation of B cells was needed. This could be achieved by different methods, but the typing results were not always reliable [9, 10]. Even with this rather low degree of reliability, the relevance of HLA-DR for solid organ transplantation and stem cells transplantation could be established [11]. The main problem remaining was the reliability of the laboratory performing the HLA-DR typing [12]. By increase of the discrepancy rate, the relevance of HLA-DR disappears [13]. The situation changed dramatically by introduction of molecular methods. The reliability of class II typing increased significantly making analyses on the relevance of class II specificities feasible.

Molecular Typing

The ability to use molecular methods and especially after standardization of the kits by the providers, typing for the class II specificities became reliable and feasible. There was no longer any need for viable cells and isolation of cells

N	77	78	79	80	81	82	83
B*3501	AGC	CTG	CGG	AAC	CTG	CGC	GGC
B*5301	A_A_C	CTG	CGG	A_T_C	G_C_G	C_T_C	_C_GC

Fig. 3. The sequence difference between HLA-B*3501 and HLA-B*5301.

expressing specific antigens. Using the polymerase chain reaction (PCR), small parts of the genome could be amplified using starters (primers) and the amplicon used for typing. The methods currently used are the following:

Sequence-specific oligonucleotide typing (SSO): This method is based on the existence of hypervariable regions within the target sequence. Probes of a rather short length (ca. 18–22 bases long) are synthesized including a dye. They can, after amplification of the target sequence, be used in a hybridization assay. Positive reactions reveal the existence of a sequence and negative reaction its missing. Simple computer programs allow the quick and (relatively) reliable definition of the specificities.

Sequence-specific priming (SSP): The method is based on the same knowledge as reported above for SSO. Instead, the target sequence is amplified and then hybridized with the specific probes, the amplification step itself then defines the specificity. A complete set of primers is used for this method. Every single specificity or a series of specificities can be defined. Positive reactions are indicated by the existence of the amplicon while negative reactions are missing.

Sequence-based typing (SBT): With this method the target sequence is directly defined using specific primers and differentially labeled bases of different chemical setup so that the elongation step is stopped after incorporation of one of these molecules (di-deoxy bases). Thus the sequence can be directly defined. Using the same example as for serology, the differences between alleles B*3501 and B*5301 are shown in figure 3.

For all these methods there is still one problem: *ambiguities*. This reflects the fact that many of the HLA alleles share sequence cassettes so that specific heterozygous combinations cannot be resolved. Additional testing is then needed. Usually this problem is not significant if one remains in homogenous populations with a rather restricted degree of polymorphism. However, typing populations with another set of HLA alleles might cause problems. The main advantage of the methods presented here, however, is the independence of viable cells. Typing can be done using different sources, like peripheral blood, spleen cells, skin, etc., in essence every DNA-carrying cell. The viability of the cells is not a limiting factor any more. Admittedly, one can state that the older the sample, the more difficult the typing. An illustration of the above said is

Table 1. A study of 740 HLA typings comparing serology and DNA methods

	Successful typing by	
	serology	DNA
Class I	45%	97%
Class II	31%	97%

depicted in table 1. Based on a total of 740 typings, we could observe that prior to the introduction of DNA typing for cornea donors of both class I and class II, the degree of typing reliability given as the percentage of successful typings was quite low (45% for class I and 31% for class II). The percentage of successful typings increased significantly to 97% for both classes after introduction of DNA typing. It is however important to decide according to the results needed which DNA typing method is suitable.

Future Perspectives

Although serological typing seems to have reached the end of the road, a great deal still has to be understood about the way HLA-specific antibodies recognize their targets. A step in this direction has been proposed by Duquesnoy [14]. His concept of three successive amino acids as the defining factor seems to be very effective. The first attempts to validate the concept have been successfully done by Witvliet et al. [15]. We need the understanding why antibodies against specific antigens are formed in order to be able to avoid sensitization of patients after solid organ transplantation.

References

1   Gorer PA: The genetic and antigenic basis of tumor transplantation. J Pathol 1937;44:691.
2   Dausset J: Leuco-agglutinins IV. Leuco-agglutinins and blood transfusion. Vox Sang 1954;4:190.
3   Van Rood JJ, van Leeuwen A, Eernisse JG: Leucocyte antibodies in sera of pregnant women, Nature 1958;181:1735.
4   Van Rood JJ: Leucocyte grouping: A method and its application; thesis, Leiden 1962.
5   Klein J, Figueroa F, Nagy ZA: Genetics of the major histocompatibility complex: The final act. Annu Rev Immunol 1983;1:119.
6   Carosella ED, Paul P, Moreau P, Rouas-Freiss N: HLA-G and HLA-E: Fundamental and pathophysiological aspects. Immunol Today 2000;21:532.
7   Terasaki PI, McClelland JD: Microdroplet assay of human serum cytotoxins. Nature 1964; 204:998.
8   Charron D (ed): Genetic Diversity of HLA: Functional and Medical Implication. Paris, EDK, 1997.

9 Verduyn W, Doxiadis IIN, Anholts J, Drabbels JJM, Naipal A, D'Amaro J, Persijn GG, Giphart MJ, Schreuder GMT: Biotinylated sequence-specific oligonucleotides: Comparison to serological HLA-DR typing of organ donors in Eurotransplant. Hum Immunol 1993;37:59–67.

10 Thorogood J, Doxiadis IIN, Schreuder GMT, van Rood JJ: Survival of serologically HLA typed and matched cadaver kidney transplants and patients: Influence of serological retyping of donors. Transplant Proc 1993;25:3051–3052.

11 Dupont B, Hansen JA: Donor selection for bone marrow transplantation: The predictive value of HLA-D typing for MLR compatibility between unrelated individuals. Transplant Proc 1978; 10:53.

12 Opelz G, Mytilineos J, Scherer S, Dunckley H, Trejaut J, Chapman J, Middleton D, Savage D, Fischer O, Bignon JD, et al: Survival of DNA HLA-DR typed and matched cadaver kidney transplants. The Collaborative Transplant Study. Lancet 1991;338:461.

13 Volker-Dieben HJ, Claas FH, Schreuder GM, Schipper RF, Pels E, Persijn GG, Smits J, D'Amaro J: Beneficial effect of HLA-DR matching on the survival of corneal allografts. Transplantation 2000;70:640.

14 Duquesnoy RJ, Marrari M: HLA matchmaker: A molecularly based algorithm for histocompatibility determination. II. Verification of the algorithm and determination of the relative immunogenicity of amino acid triplet-defined epitopes. Hum Immunol 2002;63:353.

15 Witvliet MD, Doxiadis IIN, de Fijter JW, Weimar W, Duquesnoy RJ, Claas FHJ, Schreuder GMT, de Lange P: Validation of the HLA matchmaker concept. Eur J Immunogenet 2002;29:128.

Dr. Ilias I.N. Doxiadis
Blood Transfusion and Transplantation Immunology,
Albinusdreef 2, E3-a, Postbox 9600,
NL–2300 RC Leiden (The Netherlands)
Tel. +31 71 526 3804, Fax +31 71 521 6751, E-Mail Doxiadis@LUMC.NL

Sundmacher R (ed): Adequate HLA Matching in Keratoplasty.
Dev Ophthalmol. Basel, Karger, 2003, vol 36, pp 12–21

....

Degree of Compatibility for HLA-A and -B Affects Outcome in High-Risk Corneal Transplantation

W. Houdijn Beekhuis, Marjolijn Bartels, Ilias I.N. Doxiadis,
Gabriel van Rij

The Eye Hospital, Rotterdam, Erasmus Medical Center, Rotterdam and
Department of Immunohaematology, University of Leiden, The Netherlands

Abstract

Background: HLA-A/-B matching on a split typing level is more laborious, more expensive and offers less chances for a well-fitting match than does matching on the conventional broad typing level. It is important, therefore, to investigate whether or not split matching offers advantages and would, therefore, be advisable.

Methods: 303 high-risk patients out of 2,471 keratoplasty patients from 1982 through 1996, whose histories were all followed prospectively, could be re-evaluated retrospectively according to their broad or split matching levels ('good' vs. 'moderate').

Results: Only a 'good' *split* level matching was significantly better than a 'moderate' one *in the long run* (up to 12 years). For the broad level matching this was only true for the first few years after keratoplasty.

Conclusion: If only HLA-A/-B are matched and if only results longer than 3–4 years (up to 12 years) are taken into consideration, then split level matching offers clear-cut advantages over broad level matching.

Introduction

Allograft rejection is a major cause of corneal transplant failure [1, 2]. Patients having corneal vascularization are considered to be at high risk for allograft rejection and failure as are individuals with a history of graft rejection [3–6].

Current research has identified HLA-A and -B antigens on corneal epithelium, stromal cells and corneal endothelial cells [7–9]. These HLA class I antigens have been shown to be targets for cytotoxic T cells in the process of graft rejection [10]. Although many studies have reported a beneficial effect of HLA-A and -B matching for corneal graft survival in high-risk patients, no consensus about HLA class I matching has yet been reached [11]. Theoretically, an increasing number of matched class I antigens would decrease the risk of allograft failure. Allocating donor corneas based on a 0 class I mismatch from a relatively small pool of typed donors will lead to long waiting times. Consequently, it is essential to know whether an increasing amount of matches significantly reduces the incidence of graft failure. Furthermore, with present available techniques, it is possible to perform HLA-A and -B typing more precisely on split level than broad level typing. Allocation of donor corneas based on the so-called 'split typing level' have to be shown to be beneficial, as more logistical efforts should be made with this type of allocation. The current practice at the Eye Hospital in Rotterdam is to use HLA-A- and -B-matched donor corneas based on a broad typing level for high-risk patients. This retrospective study was performed to evaluate the long-term graft survival of high-risk HLA-A- and -B-matched corneal grafts and to analyze if increasing numbers of matching or allocation based on split typing contributes to a decreased risk of immunological graft failure.

Patients and Methods

Patients

Between January 1982 and January 1996, a total of 2,471 penetrating keratoplasties (PKP) were performed at the Eye Hospital in Rotterdam. HLA-A- and -B-matched donor corneas were obtained for patients considered to be at high risk (n = 325, 13.15%) due to either previous rejected transplants or deep stromal vascularization in two or more corneal quadrants. Clinical records of all high-risk patients who received a matched corneal transplant were reviewed. Indications were classified into 14 different groups. Possible indications were anterior and stromal dystrophies, congenital malformation, keratoconus, buphthalmus, scrofulosis, leukoma or ulcer, herpes keratitis, melting diseases, Fuchs' dystrophy, (pseudophakic) bullous keratopathy, trauma, chemical or thermal burns, allograft failure and a category of 'other' indications.

All corneal grafts had to become clear after surgery and a diagnosis of immunological graft failure could not be made within a 10-day period after the transplantation. We excluded patients who were lost to follow-up within the first 2 postoperative weeks (n = 15) and patients whose transplants never became clear after PKP (n = 5). Furthermore, 2 patients were excluded as the exact HLA typing of the donor cornea could not be traced.

A total of 303 high-risk and HLA-A- and -B-matched corneal transplants met the inclusion criteria.

Methods

HLA-A and -B typing of donors and recipients was performed using the complement-dependent cytotoxicity assay at the Department of Immunohaematology and Blood Transfusion of Leiden University Medical Center, accredited by the European Federation for Immunogenetics. Analysis was performed both on the broad HLA typing level and split typing level. Donor corneas were allocated based on broad typing where more than two mismatches were not accepted. All donor corneas were obtained from Bio Implant Service (Tissue Branch of The Netherlands Transplant Foundation) and the Dutch Eye Bank, The Netherlands. All patients were treated with topical dexamethasone eyedrops (0.1%, 6 times daily) and chloramphenicol (0.5%, 3 times daily) for 2 months after transplantation. Dexamethasone eyedrops were gradually tapered off within a minimum of 1 year after the transplantation. Donor procurement and medical procedures did not change throughout the duration of the study.

Statistics

Subgroups of patients were made based on the number of HLA-A and -B mismatches for broad typing as well as for split typing. The 'good' match group was formed by patients with no or one mismatch (n = 277 with broad typing and n = 218 with split typing). The 'moderate' match group was formed by patients with two matches based on broad typing (n = 26) or by patients with two or more matches based on split typing (n = 85). Comparability of patient, donor and graft covariates between the subgroups were analyzed using the χ^2 test for categorical variables and the independent T test for continuous covariates.

Graft survival curves were made by the Kaplan-Meier method and compared with the data of the log rank test. The endpoint used was permanent immunological graft failure.

Odds ratio and adjusted survival probabilities for the different subgroups were estimated with the Cox's proportional hazards model. Variables moderately correlated to graft failure according to univariate analyses (p < 0.20) were included in the model.

Results

The median follow-up period for the 303 high-risk corneal transplants was 4.2 years. Overall graft survival is presented in figure 1. Eighty-seven percent of corneal grafts survived 1 year after transplantation and 59% survived 5 years. During the entire follow-up period, 56.5% of all corneal grafts remained functional and clear. Immune rejection was the cause of 33.3% of all graft failures. Patient, donor and graft characteristics of the total study population and the different subgroups are presented in table 1. For the subgroup based on broad matching, only the number of previous corneal transplants in the study eye differed significantly (p = 0.045), with a higher number of previous grafts found in the 'moderate' group. More patients with a history of herpes simplex keratitis were included in the 'moderate' subgroup based on split typing (p = 0.02).

We investigated the relationship of HLA matching and immunological graft failure for broad typing as well as for split typing. Considering long-term

---

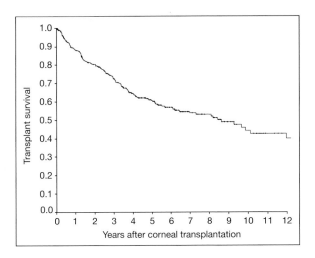

Fig. 1. Overall corneal transplant survival.

graft survival, corneal grafts with a good match based on broad typing did not have a significantly longer immunological failure-free survival compared to the group with two mismatches (log rank test p = 0.36; fig. 2). A small beneficial effect could be seen for the good match group in the first 3 years after transplantation, although this was not significant (log rank test, p = 0.09). However, when the good and moderate match group were constituted based on split typing, a significantly longer immune failure-free graft survival was found in the good match group (log rank test, p = 0.002; fig. 3). Besides matching, other factors could have influenced immunological graft failure. To correct for these possible confounding variables, we performed a multivariate analysis adjusting for variables moderately correlated with immune failure. Only the variables of indication for transplantation and number of previous grafts in the same eye were correlated (p = 0.03 and 0.001 respectively). After multivariate analyses with Cox regression methods, we also noted that a significant beneficial effect of matching could be found only if matches were calculated on the split typing level. The odds ratio (2.45) and confidence interval of the Cox regression analysis are presented in table 2. To control for the fact that there was a significantly higher number of patients with a history of HSK in the moderate group of split typing (χ^2 test, p = 0.02) and the fact that it is very difficult to differentiate between a recurrence of HSK and graft rejection, we also analyzed immune failure-free graft survival without considering patients having a history of HSK. There was a beneficial effect (log rank test, p = 0.0002) seen in the good match group based on split typing. This effect was even greater than

Table 1. Data of study group and subgroups

	Study group	Subgroup based on broad matching		Subgroup based on split matching	
		good match group	moderate match group	good match group	moderate match group
Number	303	277	26	216	87
Age, years Mean	55.8	55.7	57.3	56.5	54.0
Range	6.2–86.9	6.6–86.9	6.2–83.6	6.6–84.6	6.2–86.9
Male:female ratio	1.0:0.67	1.0:0.65	1.0:0.7	1.0:0.76	1.0:0.45
History of glaucoma, %	18.2	19.0	15.4	17.9	18.7
History of HSK	95 (31.4%)	84	11	59	36
Number of previous matched transplants (mean)	1.16	1.13	1.37	1.13	1.21
Number of previous transplants (mean)	2.28	2.22	2.70	2.28	2.25
Graft size (mm), mean	7.62	7.63	7.60	7.62	7.63

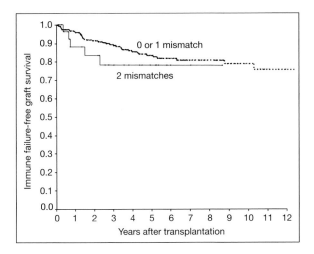

Fig. 2. Groups analyzed according to the results of *broad* matching.

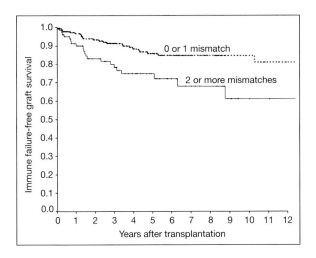

Fig. 3. Groups analyzed according to the results of *split* matching.

when considering all patients, despite the loss of power with a smaller study group (n = 208).

Finally, we analyzed the effect of HLA-A and -B split matching on immune failure-free graft survival individually, using Cox regression. According to this analysis, optimal matching (zero mismatches) at either one of these loci is signif-icantly associated with a longer immune failure-free graft survival. The benefits

Table 2. Crude and adjusted odds ratio of immunological graft failure

		Crude OR (95% CI)	OR[1] (95% CI)
Broad matching	0 or 1 mismatch	0.65 (0.25–1.65)	0.87 (0.33–2.30)
	2 mismatches		
Split matching	0 or 1 mismatch	0.41 (0.23–0.73)	0.41 (0.22–0.74)
	2 or more mismatches		

[1]Odds ratio adjusted for number of previous transplants and indication for current transplantation.

of HLA-A matching were more pronounced (p = 0.008 for split matches at HLA-A and 0.025 for split matches at HLA-B).

Discussion

The results of this study show the advantages of matching HLA-A and -B antigens using split typing for high-risk corneal transplantations. Grafts with up to one mismatch on split typing level had a significantly longer immune failure-free survival compared to grafts consisting of two or more mismatches.

Many studies suggest that HLA-A and -B matching is associated with an improved outcome of corneal graft survival in high-risk corneal transplantations [3, 12–19]. Other studies, such as the large Collaborative Corneal Transplantation Study (CCTS), fail to demonstrate a correlation of HLA matches and graft survival [11]. Most reports do not describe whether their HLA typing is based on the broad or the more precise split typing level. Current practice, when using matched donor corneas, allocates donor corneas based on broad typing [20]. Consequently, it is most likely that the majority of studies describe the influence of HLA broad matches on corneal graft survival. In this investigation however, we analyzed the influence of HLA matching on immunological graft failure on a broad typing level as well as on a split typing level. A valuable effect of HLA matching was shown only if matches were calculated based on split antigens. Analogous to this finding, a previous study showed that HLA-DR matching was beneficial for high-risk corneal transplantations only in case split antigen typing results were used [21].

Nevertheless, studies differ in their definition of high risk, consequently making it difficult to compare graft survival rates. In our study, patients were considered to be of a high risk for corneal transplant failure if they had deep stromal vascularization in two or more quadrants or if they had suffered a previous corneal graft failure due to rejection in the same eye. The CCTS included high-risk patients according to equal criteria, making it comparable to our own investigation. The overall failure rate reported by this group, using an intensive postoperative topical immunosuppressive regimen, was 35% at 3 years postoperatively. These findings are comparable to our result of 39% graft failure at 3 years.

Our survival rates compare favorably with other studies, despite the inclusion of all risk categories in these studies [22]. One third of graft failures in our study are due to an irreversible rejection reaction. Previous investigators reported similar results, showing that allograft rejection is still the leading cause of corneal graft failure [22, 23]. Overall graft survival depends also on the presence of non-immunological factors causing graft failure, such as improvement of surgical techniques [24, 25], training of corneal surgeons [26] or the use of newer topical or systemic immunosuppressive medication [27–29].

Although this study was performed retrospectively, we were not aware of the number of HLA matches at the time of diagnosing the final graft outcome, because these data were kept in a separate data file. The diagnosis of an immune mediated graft failure is not always clear-cut. A rejection reaction and recurrence of HSK can be especially difficult to distinguish clinically, more so during our investigation as this differentiation had to be made retrospectively. To obviate this problem, we analyzed solely the influence of HLA-A and -B matches by excluding patients with a history of HSK in the study eye. This analysis showed the same beneficial results for the good match group based on split typing.

The good and moderate match subgroups were comparable with respect to most characteristics mentioned in table 2. However, a higher number of previous grafts was observed in the moderate match group based on broad typing. This variable was a risk factor for immunological graft failure, which explains the difference between the crude and adjusted (including this variable in the model) odds ratio for the subgroups based on broad typing. Furthermore, more patients with a HSK were included in the moderate match group based on split typing, however, analysis of immune failure-free graft survival without considering these patients showed the same results.

In conclusion, one third of the graft failures of our investigated high-risk corneal transplantations were due to an irreversible graft rejection. This number could possibly be lowered by allocating donor corneas based on split antigen matching since HLA-A and -B matching on the split antigen level contributes to a higher immune failure-free graft survival.

References

1   Vail A, Gore SM, Bradley BA, et al: Conclusions of the corneal transplant follow-up study. Br J Ophthalmol 1997;81:631–636.
2   Khodadoust AA: The allograft rejection reaction: The leading cause of late failure of clinical corneal grafts; in Corneal Graft Failure. Ciba Found Symp. Amsterdam, Elsevier, 1973, pp 51–167.
3   Völker-Dieben HJ, Kok-van Alphen CC, Lansbergen Q, et al: The effect of prospective HLA-A and -B matching on corneal graft survival. Acta Ophthalmol 1982;60:203–212.
4   Williams KA, Roder D, Esterman A, et al: Factors predictive of corneal graft survival. Ophthalmology 1992;99:403–444.
5   Boisjoly HM, Tourigny R, Bazir R, et al: Risk factors of corneal graft failure. Ophthalmology 1993;11:1728–1735.
6   Völker-Dieben HJ, Kok-van Alphen CC, Lansbergen Q, et al: Different influence on corneal graft survival in 539 transplants. Acta Ophthalmol 1982;60:190–202.
7   Pels E, Van der Gaag R: HLA-A, -B, -C and HLA-DR antigens and dendritic cells in fresh and organ-cultured preserved corneas. Cornea 1985;3:231–239.
8   Whitsett CF, Stulting RD: The distribution of HLA antigens on human corneal tissue. Invest Ophthalmol Vis Sci 1984;25:519–524.
9   Li Q, He Y: An immunohistochemical study of Langerhans cells, T cells and the HLA antigen in human cornea. Yen Ko Hsueh Pao 1993;19:121–125.
10   Roelen DL, van Beelen E, van Bree SP, et al: The presence of activated donor HLA class I-reactive T lymphocytes is associated with rejection of corneal grafts. Transplantation 1995;59: 1039–1042.
11   Collaborative Corneal Transplantation Studies: Effectiveness of histocompatibility matching in high-risk corneal transplantation. Arch Ophthalmol 1992;110:1392–1403.
12   Foulks GN, Sanfillipo F: Beneficial effects of histocompatibility in high-risk corneal transplantation. Am J Ophthalmol 1982;94:622–629.
13   Sanfilippo F, MacQueen JM, Vaughn WK, et al: Reduced graft rejection with good HLA-A and -B matching in high-risk corneal transplantation. N Engl J Med 1986;315:29–35.
14   Boisjoly HM, Roy R, Bernard PM, et al: Association between corneal allograft rejections and HLA compatibility. Ophthalmology 1990;12:1689–1698.
15   Ozdemir O: A prospective study of histocompatibility testing for keratoplasty in high-risk patients. Br J Ophthalmol 1986;70:183–186.
16   Batchelor JR, Casey TA, Gibbs DC, et al: HLA matching and corneal grafting. Lancet 1976;i: 551–554.
17   Morita N, Munkhbat B, Kanai N, et al: Effect of HLA-A and -DPB1 matching in corneal transplantation. Transplant Proc 1998;30:3491–3492.
18   Munkhbath B, Hagihara M, Sato T, et al: HLA class II DNA typing using ocular tissue and its usefulness in corneal transplantation. Transplant Proc 1996;3:1257–1258.
19   Vail A, Gore SM, Bradley BA, et al: Influence of donor and histocompatibility factors on corneal graft outcome. Transplantation 1994;58:1210–1216.
20   Völker-Dieben HJ, Claas FHJ, Schreuder GMT, et al: Beneficial effect of HLA-DR matching on the survival of corneal allografts. Transplantation 2000;4:640–648.
21   Bartels MC, Otten HG, van Gelderen BE, Van der Lelij A: Influence of HLA-A, HLA-B and HLA-DR matching on rejection of random corneal grafts using corneal tissue for retrospective DNA HLA typing. Br J Ophthalmol 2001;85:1341–1346.
22   Vail A, Gore SM, Bradley BA, et al: Corneal graft survival and visual outcome: A multicentre study. Ophthalmology 1994;101:120–127.
23   Williams KA, Muehlberg SM, Lewis RF, et al: The Australian Corneal Graft Registry 1996 Report. Adelaide, Mercury Press, 1997, p 19.
24   Christo CG, Van Rooy J, Geerards AJ, Remeyer L, Beekhuis WH: Suture-related complications following keratoplasty: A 5-year retrospective study. Cornea 2001;20:816–819.
25   Melles GR, Remeyer L, Geerards AJ, Beekhuis WH: The future of lamellar keratoplasty. Curr Opin Ophthalmol 1999;10:253–259.

26   Waldock A, Cook SD: Corneal transplantation: How successful are we? Br J Ophthalmol 2000;84: 813–815.
27   Hill JC: Systemic cyclosporin in high-risk keratoplasties: Short- versus long-term therapy. Ophthalmology 1994;101:128–133.
28   Hikita N, Lopez JS, Chan CC, et al: Use of topical FK-506 in a corneal graft rejection model in Lewis rats. Invest Ophthalmol Vis Sci 1997;38:901–909.
29   Lam DSC, Wong AKK, Tham CCY, et al: The use of combined intravenous pulse methylprednisolone and oral cyclosporin A in the treatment of corneal graft rejection: A preliminary study. Eye 1998;12:615–618.

W.H. Beekhuis
Cornea Service, The Eye Hospital Rotterdam,
180 Schiedamse Vest, NL–3011 BH Rotterdam (The Netherlands)
Tel. +31 10 401 7740, Fax +31 10 213 3336, E-Mail hi.beekhuis@planet.nl

Sundmacher R (ed): Adequate HLA Matching in Keratoplasty.
Dev Ophthalmol. Basel, Karger, 2003, vol 36, pp 22–41

....

Histocompatibility and Corneal Transplantation

H.J. Völker-Dieben[a], *G.M.Th. Schreuder*[b], *F.H.J. Claas*[b], *I.I.N. Doxiadis*[b],
R.F. Schipper[c], *E. Pels*[d], *G.G. Persijn*[e], *J. Smits*[e], *J. D'Amaro*[b]

[a]Department of Ophthalmology, Vrije Universiteit Medisch Centrum, Amsterdam;
[b]Department of Immunohematology and Blood Transfusion, Leiden University
Medical Center, Leiden; [c]Supervisory Organization for Health Insurance,
Amstelveen; [d]The Netherlands Ophthalmic Research Institute, Amsterdam,
and [e]The Eurotransplant Foundation, Leiden, The Netherlands

Abstract

Background: HLA typing and matching have been poorly implemented in corneal
transplantation, mainly because of inconclusive or contradictory analytical results.
Consequently, we studied the immune response of corneal transplant recipients to HLA
histoincompatibilities in a large homogeneous study.

Methods: All corneal transplantations were performed by a single surgeon in a single
center between 1976 and 1996. Population genetic and other statistical analyses were performed. Simulation studies assessed the effects of HLA-DR mistypings on analytical results.

Results: Mono- and multivariate analyses identified retransplantation, degree of vascularization, HLA-AB and -DR match grades, endothelial cell count, graft size, recipient
gender, storage method and panel-reactive antibodies as significantly influencing the survival of corneal transplants. Simulation studies showed that the beneficial effect of HLA-DR
matching is abrogated by HLA-DR mistypings.

Conclusions: Corneal transplant recipients have a normal immune response to HLA
incompatibilities. Demonstration of that fact requires accurate HLA typings.

Introduction

In 1943, Gibson and Medawar [1] showed that second skin transplants from
the same human donors were rejected more rapidly than first grafts. In 1946,

Medawar [2] demonstrated the homology between tissue and leukocyte antigens. He showed that the rejection of skin transplants in rabbits was significantly accelerated when preceded by a previous skin transplant or by the injection of leukocytes.

It was not until 1962 that the first di-allelic human leukocyte group system, 4a and 4b, was described [3]. In subsequent years, knowledge of human leukocyte antigens has progressed to the state where many antigenic determinants controlled by multiple closely linked complex loci can be recognized by serologic and/or molecular techniques.

Similar studies in other vertebrate species have demonstrated the presence of clusters of genes on a single chromosomal segment that control similar antigens and other immunologically interrelated functions. Those genes constitute the major histocompatibility complex (MHC) of the species.

Frelinger and Shreffler [4] have listed the following common features of MHCs: (1) principal transplantation barrier of the species; (2) serologically detected antigens of lymphocytes, broadly distributed on other tissues; (3) major factors which stimulate mixed leukocyte reaction (MLR) and graft-versus-host reaction (GVHR); (4) immune response genes; resistance to disease; (5) multiple phenotypic traits or functions controlled by a tight cluster of multiple genetic loci, and (6) extensive genetic polymorphism at many loci in the complex.

The driving force behind the identification of the human major histocompatibility locus (HLA) was the search for polymorphic antigens to be used to match donors with recipients for transplantation.

There is nothing in the definition of MHCs that justifies the exclusion of corneal tissue from its effects. Nevertheless, that erroneous assumption has been accepted by some investigators since they were not able to demonstrate a beneficial HLA matching effect.

HLA typing and matching have been used for more than four decades for solid organ transplantations. However, that practice has not yet achieved universal acceptance for cornea transplantation, mainly because of inconclusive or contradictory analytical results [5–29].

Van Rood et al. [30] cited four possible reasons for disparate results in kidney transplantation follow-up studies: (1) poor quality HLA typing negates the effect of matching; (2) when the number of good (or poor) matches is low, a matching effect is not demonstrable; (3) aggressive immunotherapy might diminish the influence of HLA matching on graft survival (however, at the cost of other complications such as malignancies [31, 32]), and (4) racial heterogeneity can make it impossible to obtain good matches.

We avoided the adverse effects of those factors by performing a comprehensive study of the immune response to HLA-A, -B and -DR histoincompatibilities in 1,681 consecutive recipients of penetrating keratoplasties which were performed by a single surgeon, in a single center, over a 20-year period, 1976–1996 [33].

Materials and Methods

Patients, HLA typings and their quality control, HLA-A, -B and -DR matching of recipients and donors, population genetics validation of HLA typing results, storage and quality control of donor corneas, clinical diagnostic criteria of graft rejection, post-operative follow-up and therapy, and data handling and statistical methods have been described previously. We also performed simulation studies to demonstrate the effects of mistyped recipient and donor HLA-DR typings on analytical results [33].

Irreversible immunological rejections constituted 41% of the causes of failure in our results. The non-immunological causes included glaucoma, recurrent herpes simplex virus infection, insufficient donor material, bacterial infections, secondary endothelial dystrophy and trauma. Cases with such failures were censored, i.e. excluded, from the analyses.

Survival curves were calculated using the actuarial life table method [34]. The significance of differences between classes was assessed with a χ^2 statistic derived from a log-rank test [35]. Relative risk (RR) estimates were derived from the values in the log-rank tables.

The absence of any rejection episode, reversible or irreversible, is a more sensitive and appropriate indicator of the immune competence of corneal transplant recipients than the time to irreversible immunological rejection that is really an indication of the efficacy of follow-up procedures, especially the immunosuppressive therapy protocols, of transplantation centers. However, since that indicator is not used universally, we have performed all of our major analyses using both indicators to enable investigators to compare their results with ours, irrespective of the end-point indicator that they use.

A Cox proportional hazards model was used for the multivariate analyses. Failures due to non-immunological causes were censored in the statistical analyses [36].

For a recent review of the essentials of HLA typing and the procedures for validating its results, see Schreuder [37] and Schipper and D'Amaro [38].

Results

Precision of HLA-DR Typings

In 1986, the HLA typing laboratory which performed all of our recipient and donor typings compared its results for 964 donor HLA-DR typings, which had been obtained with a serological cytotoxicity test using an HLA-DR serum set provided by Eurotransplant and/or local sera, with the results which it had obtained by using a PCR-biotin-SSO technique which was performed on the mononuclear cells from donor spleen samples. Those results revealed a concordance rate for the serological and molecular HLA-DR typings of

90.8% [39]. In 1997, the concordance rate for 382 HLA-DR retypings was 99.2% [40].

We used population genetic analytical techniques to confirm the results of the periodic quality assurance studies that are carried out regularly to assess the precision of the HLA typings. The goodness-of-fit tests for Hardy-Weinberg equilibrium for the HLA-A, -B and -DR loci were used to assess if the numbers of different phenotype combinations in those loci agreed with the numbers predicted by the gene frequencies of the HLA alleles in those loci [41, 42]. The test result p values were all clearly above the minimum significance level of 0.05. For the recipient typings, the p values were 0.385 for HLA-A, 0.111 for HLA-B and 0.906 for HLA-DR. For the donor typings, the p values were 0.747 for HLA-A, 0.116 for HLA-B and 0.833 for HLA-DR.

The HLA gene frequencies in the donor and recipient populations were similar to each other and to those in a healthy Dutch Caucasoid control population. Those precise typing results were not surprising since the same experienced laboratory typed all of those individuals, but they nevertheless demonstrate the consistency and reliability of the typing results that formed the basis for assigning the match grades that were used to pair donors with recipients.

Identification of Factors That Exert a Beneficial Effect on the Survival of Corneal Transplants

Monovariate Analyses

Monovariate analyses of high-risk cases, i.e. those with recipient corneal vascularization in 2 or more quadrants, were used to identify the factors that exerted a significant beneficial effect on the survival of corneal transplants. The actuarial survival curve analyses were performed twice. Their results are shown only for the significant factors. The following additional factors were tried also but their results were not significant: blood transfusion history; recipient and donor ABO blood groups, and age.

HLA-A, -B Matching: Only Irreversible Immunological Rejection Episodes

The first set of survival curve analyses used only the high-risk cases whose cause of failure was only an irreversible immunological rejection event (table 1). The Kaplan-Meier estimates of the cumulative proportion of corneal grafts

Table 1. Results of monovariate analyses; failure is irreversible immunological rejection only

Factor	log-rank p value	% clear grafts at 5 years	Cases[a]
Retransplantation: yes/no	0.024	77/85	388/463
Vascularization: high/low risk[b]	<0.000001	81/94	851/530
HLA-A, -B mism: 3–4/0–2 (see fig. 1)	0.00003	67/85	207/642
HLA-DR mism: 1–2/0 (see fig. 2)	0.005	83/97	214/066
Cell count: <2,000 mm^2/≥2,000 mm^2	0.003	75/85	298/553
Graft size: ≥8.0 mm/<8.0 mm	0.004	68/84	144/707
Recipient gender: male/female	0.051	77/85	436/415
Organ culture storage: no/yes	0.003	74/84	267/584

mism = Mismatches; p value = significance of the difference between the 2 survival curves.

[a]Cases: For transplant number, 388/463 indicates 388 cases who were retransplanted and 463 cases who received only 1 transplant. A similar interpretation should be used for the cases listed for the other factors.

[b]No selection for vascularization risk status. All cases analyzed.

which failed due to only irreversible immunological events are displayed in figure 1 for the 642 HLA-AB matched and 207 AB mismatched cases: 85.3% at 5 years for the 0–2 AB mismatched cases and 67.4% at 5 years for the 3–4 AB mismatched cases, p value by log-rank test = 0.00003. The RR of failure for the 3–4 AB mismatched cases versus the 0–2 AB mismatched cases was 2.73, p < 0.0001.

HLA-DR Matching: Only Irreversible Immunological Rejection Episodes

The Kaplan-Meier estimates of the cumulative proportion of corneal grafts which failed due to only irreversible immunological rejection events are displayed in figure 2 for the 66 HLA-DR matched and 214 DR mismatched cases: 97.1% at 5 years for the 0 DR mismatched cases and 82.7% at 5 years for the 1–2 DR mismatched cases, p value by log-rank test = 0.005. The RR of failure for the 1–2 DR mismatched cases versus the 0 DR mismatched cases was 8.06, p = 0.005 (table 1).

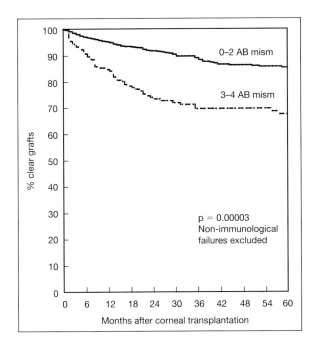

Fig. 1. Influence of HLA-AB matching on high-risk corneal transplants. *Only irreversible immunological rejections* were analyzed. *High-risk* recipients are those with *moderate* or *severe* pre-operative corneal vascularization in 2 or more quadrants.

Cases at risk at 6 month intervals after cornea transplantation:

Curve	0	6	12	18	24	30	36	42	48	54	60
0–2 AB mism	642	573	503	451	405	366	325	287	255	231	195
3–4 AB mism	207	167	139	121	103	85	71	64	57	51	48

HLA-A, -B Matching: All Immunological Rejection Episodes

The second set of survival curve analyses used our entire data set of high-risk recipients and their donors. All immunological events, reversible or irreversible, were analyzed (table 2). The Kaplan-Meier estimates of the cumulative proportion of corneal grafts which failed due to any immunological event are displayed in figure 3 for the 642 HLA-AB matched and 207 AB mismatched cases: 75.2% at 5 years for the 0–2 AB mismatched cases and 57.7% at 5 years for the 3–4 AB mismatched cases, p value by log-rank test = 0.0004. The RR of failure for the 3–4 AB mismatched cases versus the 0–2 AB mismatched cases was 2.09, p = 0.0001.

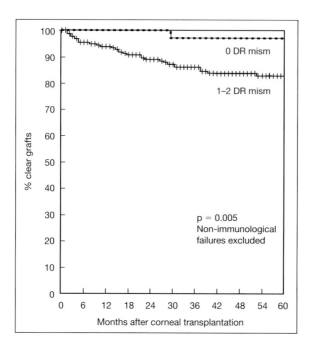

Fig. 2. Influence of HLA-DR matching on high-risk corneal transplants. *Only irre-versible immunological rejections* were analyzed. *High-risk* recipients are those with *moderate* or *severe* pre-operative corneal vascularization in 2 or more quadrants.

Cases at risk at 6 month intervals after cornea transplantation:

Curve	0	6	12	18	24	30	36	42	48	54	60
0 DR mism	66	60	50	46	36	28	21	17	15	12	10
1–2 DR mism	214	192	167	148	138	123	107	90	82	71	62

HLA-DR Matching: All Immunological Rejection Episodes

The Kaplan-Meier estimates of the cumulative proportion of corneal grafts which failed due to any immunological event are displayed in figure 4 for the 66 HLA-DR matched and 214 DR mismatched cases: 84.8% at 5 years for the 0 DR mismatched cases and 71.4% at 5 years for the 1–2 DR mismatched cases, p value by log-rank test = 0.040. The RR of failure for the 1–2 DR mismatched cases versus the 0 DR mismatched cases was 2.39, p = 0.024 (table 2).

Table 2. Results of monovariate analyses; failure is any immunological rejection episode, reversible or irreversible

Factor	log-rank p value	% clear grafts at 5 years	Cases[a]
Vascularization: high/low risk[b]	<0.000001	71/89	851/830
HLA-A, -B mism: 3–4/0–2 (see fig. 3)	0.0004	58/75	207/642
HLA-DR mism: 1–2/0 (see fig. 4)	0.040	71/85	214/066
Graft size: ≥8.0 mm/<8.0 mm	0.006	54/74	144/707
Recipient gender: male/female	0.032	66/76	436/415

mism = Mismatches; p value = significance of the difference between the 2 curves.
[a]Cases: For vascularization, 851/830 indicates 851 high-risk cases and 830 low-risk cases. A similar interpretation should be used for the cases listed for the other factors.
[b]No selection for vascularization risk status. All cases analyzed.

Joint Effect of HLA-A, -B and -DR Matching

The hypothesis for a joint effect of HLA-A, -B and -DR matching was supported by the fact that, among the 553 cases that were typed for those three loci, 7 grafts with 0 DR mismatches but 1 or 2 AB mismatches failed and 8 grafts with 0 AB mismatches but 1 DR mismatch failed. A similar observation was made in 1986 by Boisjoly et al. [43].

Multivariate Analyses on the Effect of HLA Matching
on the Survival of Corneal Transplants

The hypothesis of an effect of MHC class I, HLA-A, -B and MHC class II, HLA-DR mismatches on corneal graft survival was tested in a stratified Cox model using a backwards selection procedure based on the likelihood ratio test. Four analyses were performed.

The first analysis used only the *time to irreversible immunological rejection* as the entry time. The final Cox proportional hazards model identified HLA-DR matching, % panel-reactive antibodies, retransplantation, HLA-AB matching, number of immunological rejection events, (reversible or irreversible), and vascularization risk class. Its results and their significance (p < 0.000001) are set out in table 3 (p. 32).

The second analysis used the *time to any immunological rejection event*, reversible or irreversible, as the entry time. We modeled the following clinically

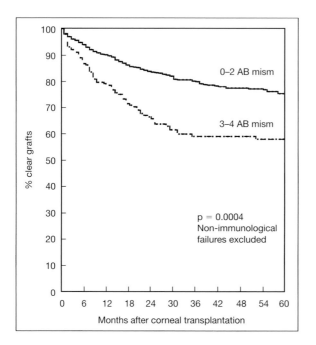

Fig. 3. Influence of HLA-AB matching on high-risk corneal transplants. *All immuno-logical rejections*, reversible or irreversible, were analyzed. *High-risk* recipients are those with *moderate* or *severe* pre-operative corneal vascularization in 2 or more quadrants.

Cases at risk at 6 month intervals after cornea transplantation:

Curve	0	6	12	18	24	30	36	42	48	54	60
0–2 AB mism	642	603	551	505	463	420	378	330	292	262	229
3–4 AB mism	207	175	150	132	117	100	89	80	71	66	59

relevant factors: time, degree of vascularization, retransplantation, number of HLA-AB and -DR mismatches, proportion of panel-reactive antibodies and number of immunological rejection events. Recipient and donor gender, endothelial cell count, storage medium, graft size, recipient and donor ABO blood groups and age were also tried but they did not make any significant contribution to the models. The results of the final Cox proportional hazards model that identified vascularization risk class, and HLA-AB and HLA-DR match grades, and their significance ($p < 0.000001$) are set out in table 4 (p. 32).

The third and fourth analyses were similar to the first and second with the addition of stratification for the four consecutive 5-year intervals covered by

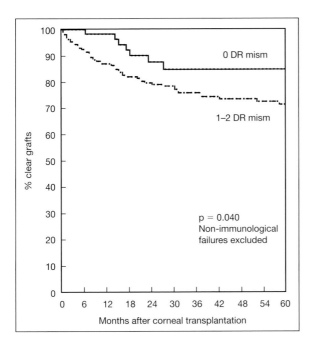

Fig. 4. Influence of HLA-DR matching on high-risk corneal transplants. *All immunological rejections*, reversible or irreversible, were analyzed. *High-risk* recipients are those with *moderate* or *severe* pre-operative corneal vascularization in 2 or more quadrants.

Cases at risk at 6 month intervals after cornea transplantation:

Curve	0	6	12	18	24	30	36	42	48	54	60
0 DR mism	66	63	55	51	43	35	26	19	17	14	12
1–2 DR mism	214	200	185	169	159	140	126	108	99	87	79

our 20-year study. Their results were not appreciably different to those in the first two analyses. They demonstrated that the performance of our Center was consistent over those two decades (data not shown).

Simulation Studies to Assess the Effect of Imprecise HLA-DR Typings

The monovariate analyses of our corneal transplant results revealed a significant beneficial effect of HLA-A, -B and -DR matching (tables 1–4, fig. 1–4). Our results were markedly different from those in the report of the CCTS study [15]. The high degree of reproducibility of our donor and recipient HLA-DR typings made us realize that we could use our well-typed HLA-DR typing results

Table 3. Results from the Cox proportional hazards model; censoring indicator variable is *irreversible immunological rejection* (455 observations)

Variable	Subset	Hazard	p value
HLA-DR mismatches	1–2/0	4.84	0.033
Panel-reactive antibodies, %	>9%/0–9%	3.54	0.004
Retransplantation	yes/no	3.26	0.002
HLA-A, -B mismatches	3–4/0–2	3.15	0.026
Number of rejection events	1–4/0	2.91	0.004
Degree of vascularization	High/low	2.84	0.025

Likelihood ratio test: 40.4041, DF = 6, p value < 0.000001.

Table 4. Results from the Cox proportional hazards model; censoring indicator variable is *any immunological rejection event – reversible or irreversible* (544 observations)

Variable	Subset	Hazard	p value
Degree of vascularization	High/low	3.25	<0.001
HLA-A, -B mismatches	3–4/0–2	2.16	0.008
HLA-DR mismatches	1–2/0	1.97	0.027

Likelihood ratio test: 36.6135, DF = 3, p value < 0.000001.

to demonstrate the effect of typing errors on analytical results which are obtained from imprecise typing data. Our goal was to determine if the results of the CCTS study could have been caused by their reported serious level of HLA-DR typing discrepancies, which was almost 40% in their recipients who had only a single reported HLA-DR antigen [44]. To achieve that goal, we randomly introduced HLA-DR typing errors of 5–40% into the HLA-DR typing results of our 280 high-risk recipients and their donors in our data file. We examined the influence of those errors on the demonstrated significant beneficial effect of HLA-DR matching (tables 1, 2, fig. 2, 4). This simulation approach is not dependent on any particular typing technique since it simply uses the phenotype assignments that were based on typing results.

When the censoring indicator variable was only irreversible immunological rejection events, the difference between the proportion of surviving grafts in the HLA-DR mismatch classes (0 and 1–2 DR mismatches), 5 years after

Table 5. Results of simulation studies of the effect of five different levels of imprecise HLA-DR typings on corneal graft survival at 5 years after transplantation

	Irreversible rejections only			All rejection episodes		
	% clear grafts		p value	% clear grafts		p value
% errors	0 DR mism	1–2 DR mism		0 DR mism	1–2 DR mism	
0	97	83	0.005	85	71	0.024
5	89	84	0.070	79	73	0.607
10	88	85	0.216	73	75	0.793
20	84	86	0.988	67	77	0.205
30	82	88	0.616	65	80	0.038
40	80	90	0.098	66	81	0.028

mism = Mismatches; p value = by the log-rank test for the significance of the difference between the 2 survival curves, for 0 and 1–2 DR mismatches, at 5 years.

transplantation, was reduced from 16% in the results from the good DR typing data to 5% when 5% errors had been introduced, and the previously highly significant result (p = 0.005) was no longer significant (p = 0.070). When 20% or more errors had been introduced, the 1–2 DR mismatched curve rose above the 0 DR curve by 2–10% (left side of table 5).

When the censoring indicator variable was any immunological rejection event, 5 years after transplantation, the difference between the proportions of surviving grafts in the HLA-DR mismatch classes (0 and 1–2 DR mismatches) was reduced from 14% in the results from the good DR typing data to 6% when 5% errors had been introduced, and the previously significant result (p = 0.024) was no longer significant (p = 0.607). When 10% or more errors were introduced, the 1–2 DR mismatched curve rose above the 0 DR curve by 2–15%. When more than 20% errors were introduced, the survival curves reached low levels of significance (p = 0.038 for the 30% error cases and p = 0.028 for the 40% error cases) (right side of table 5).

Irrespective of the censoring indicator variable which was used (only irreversible immunological rejection or any immunological rejection event, reversible or irreversible), the results with those simulated imprecisely typed recipients led to overestimates of the number of mismatches. Their results improved the performance of 1–2 DR mismatch class, by 7% (from 83 to 90%) when only irreversible immunological rejections were analyzed, and

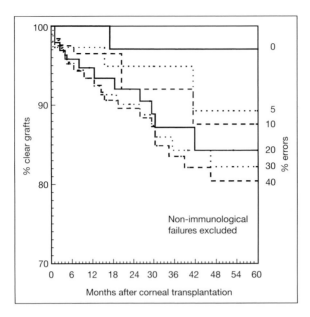

Fig. 5. Effect of inducing 5–40% HLA-DR typing errors into 280 precise DR typings on the results of corneal transplant survival analyses. Part 1. Results for cases reassigned into the 0 DR mismatched class. Results of a simulation study.

10% (from 71 to 81%) when all immunological rejections were analyzed (table 5, fig. 6).

Imprecisely typed donors lead to underestimates of the number of mismatches and the assignment of those cases to the 0 DR mismatch class. Consequently, the performance of that mismatched class is reduced, by 17% (from 97 to 80%) when only irreversible immunological rejections were analyzed, and 19% (from 85 to 66%) when all immunological rejections were analyzed (table 5, fig. 5).

The combined effect of the imprecise typings is seen as an alterations in the difference between the proportion of surviving grafts in the 2 HLA-DR mismatch classes (0 and 1–2 DR mismatches). The previous degree of separation between their respective survival curves is initially reduced and finally the proportions may be reversed with the curve for the 1–2 mismatched cases lying above the curve for the well-matched 0 mismatched cases (table 5).

The post-transplant histories of corneal transplant recipients provide us with compelling evidence of the importance of histocompatibility factors for the survival of those transplants, namely 450 *recipients*, 27% of our 1,681 recipients had reversible or irreversible immunological rejection episodes. The efficacy of our immunosuppression therapy protocol was demonstrated by

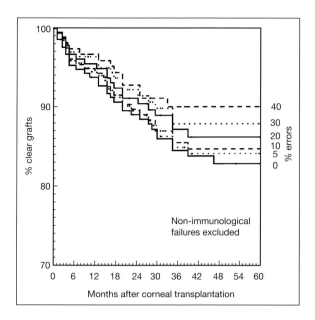

Fig. 6. Effect of inducing 5–40% HLA-DR typing errors into 280 precise DR typings on the results of corneal transplant survival analyses. Part 2. Results for cases reassigned into the 1–2 DR mismatched class. Results of a simulation study.

the fact that only 14% of the cases that had a reversible rejection episode were followed ultimately by an irreversible immunological rejection.

Discussion

Our single-center studies avoided potential 'center effect' factors that could have influenced our results [45]. The results of our mono- and multivariate analyses reveal that corneal transplant recipients have a normal immune response to HLA histoincompatibilities.

There were clear differences between our results and those that were reported on a multi-center, multi-surgeon study by the Collaborative Corneal Transplant Study Group (CCTS) [15]. The authors of that report concluded that for high-risk patients who are immunosuppressed by topical steroid therapy, neither HLA-A, -B nor HLA-DR antigen matching substantially reduced the likelihood of corneal graft failure, that a positive donor-recipient cross-match did not increase the risk of corneal graft failure and that ABO blood group matching may be effective in reducing the risk of graft failure due to irreversible immunological rejection.

Their results clearly contradicted other reports of a clear-cut significant beneficial effect of HLA-A, -B and HLA-DR matching. They commented in their report that 'A beneficial effect of HLA matching on graft survival may have been abrogated in the CCTS by postoperative steroid therapy'. However, such a practice may increase the possibility of complications like glaucoma, cataracts, infections, delayed wound healing, wound dehiscence and malignancies.

They also mentioned that the degree of histocompatibility matching/mismatching may not have been accurately assessed in their donor and recipient populations because of their ethnic diversity. That is a possibility that occurs more frequently than is recognized. The mobility of diverse populations and the increasing number of refugees that are granted asylum in 'foreign' countries exacerbates the problem.

Examination of the Joint Report of the Fifth Histocompatibility Workshop revealed that serum reports by the reference laboratories demonstrated a considerable amount of variation in the reactivity of groups of antisera against single antigenic specificities. Sera that were well defined in European and North American Caucasoids reacted similarly as well-defined clusters when they were tested in those populations, but they did not do so when they were tested in non-Caucasoid populations [46]. For example, 5 anti-HLA-A10 sera gave highly correlated concordant results in Caucasoid populations but their results in the Oceanian populations suggested that those same sera were reacting against multiple antigenic variants that were not present in Caucasoid populations [47].

The publication of a report by the CCTS study group on the reproducibility of their HLA-A, -B and -DR typings revealed a possible explanation of their results [44]. They performed those studies because they observed that the level of homozygosity, i.e. the proportion of cases with only one antigen in a single HLA locus, was more than twice the expected level for the HLA-DR locus. They retyped 129 patients with less than 2 DR antigens. The concordance between the original and retypings was 55% for HLA-DR, and it rose to 59% when they excluded the antigens that were difficult to type. The most common error that they identified was the failure to identify a second DR locus antigen.

The total magnitude of typing errors in their study is unknown, since none of the remaining patients and none of the donors were retyped. However, our simulation studies, which introduced similar HLA-DR typing errors into our 280 well-typed patient and donor HLA-DR typings, showed that even small amounts of imprecise HLA-DR typings, as little as 5% can abrogate the true beneficial effect of HLA-DR matching on the survival of corneal transplants and that larger amounts of imprecise typings can lead to an apparent adverse effect of HLA-DR matching as shown in the results of the CCTS study [3] and in reports on the negative effect of HLA-DR matching on corneal graft rejection from the UK [16–18].

So far, we have observed only a single irreversible immunological graft rejection in the 66 high-risk cases with 0 HLA-DR mismatches. That 82-year-old male patient had a single HLA-A locus mismatch, A2, and no HLA-B, -C or -DR mismatches. He was successfully treated for a rejection episode that occurred 16 months after transplantation. Fourteen months later, he had an irreversible immunological rejection. Prior to that event, he had no detectable HLA antibodies in his serum. One week later, an anti-HLA-A2 antibody was detected in his serum. That case is a good example of a normal immune response to an HLA histoincompatibility in an elderly corneal transplant recipient [23].

The significant beneficial effect of HLA-A, -B and -DR typing and matching on the survival of high-risk corneal transplants justifies that practice for all high-risk recipients of corneal transplants. The joint effect of HLA-A, -B and -DR matching which we and others have found suggests that attempts must be made to minimize the number of mismatches by typing and matching recipients and donors for the antigens at those 3 loci.

Although there is a strong significant association between the degree of corneal vascularization and the survival of corneal transplants, that factor, per se, is not the underlying reason. We have found no significant correlation between the time to onset of rejection episodes and degrees of vascularization, i.e. in high- and low-risk cases. The explanation for that association is more complex.

The presence of HLA-A, -B and -DR and minor H antigens in the cornea makes it vulnerable to the immune response of immunocompetent graft recipients [8, 48, 49]. However, antigenic challenges do not readily lead to immune responses in the ocular environment as compared to other anatomical sites, but rather lead to tolerance [50]. Antigens that are delivered via the blood-vascular route induce immune deviation and down-regulation, rather than activation, of cell-mediated immune responses [51].

Niederkorn [52] has suggested that the association between the degree of corneal vascularization and the increased risk for corneal graft rejection involve changes in the corneal graft bed that are caused by stimuli that evoke neovascularization – like viral and bacterial infections, trauma, phagocytic stimuli and the transplantation process itself, i.e. sutures and cautery. Those factors also stimulate the migration and accumulation of antigen-presenting Langerhans' cells (LCs) in the corneal epithelium that lead to the activation of T cells and subsequent transplant rejection [53, 54] and the appearance of lymphatic vessels. The induction of LCs and lymphatics, rather than the presence of blood vessels, may be the crucial factors responsible for abolishing the immune privilege of the corneal graft bed.

Mismatched HLA class I antigens (HLA-A and -B) are believed to be the main targets for cytotoxic T lymphocytes and alloantibodies. HLA class II (HLA-DR) mismatches lead to the activation of the regulatory T lymphocytes of the recipient. The presence of donor-specific HLA alloantibodies [5] and cytotoxic T lymphocytes [6] on rejected corneal transplants supports the hypothesis that HLA matching is involved in the rejection process. LCs are found in the peripheral region of the corneal epithelium. Those cells or their precursors are the only epidermal cells expressing HLA class II antigens or their equivalents [7]. HLA-DR-positive LCs are found in the central corneal epithelium of rejected transplants and in herpetic corneas. They are found only in the limbus of healthy corneas [8, 51].

Donor corneas that are stored for 14 days in organ culture are negative for HLA-DR-positive LCs [9]. The higher proportion of transplant rejection episodes in larger grafts than in smaller ones (tables 1, 2) may be attributed to the presence of LCs that express HLA class I and II antigens. The afferent blockade of the immune response can be bypassed by donor-derived LCs. Those cells serve as potent immunogens for all categories of corneal transplants except those that only involve disparity at the HLA-A, -B locus [10, 11].

Long-term clear grafts may be rejected after they become vascularized as a consequence of trauma, bacterial or viral infections. Inflammatory factors may induce the expression of HLA-DR molecules on the corneal endothelium [12, 55, 56]. Consequently, all recipients, especially the younger ones who obviously will have a longer period of exposure to such factors than elderly recipients, should also receive HLA matched grafts, irrespective of the degree of vascularization of their corneas at the time of transplantation. However, the implementation of such a policy is feasible only when there is an adequate supply of donor corneas for matching purposes.

HLA typing and matching procedures, which are used for solid organs and other tissues, should also be applied in corneal transplantation. The disparity in the published reports on the differential survival of corneal transplants in HLA-A, -B and -DR matched and unmatched donor/recipient pairs may have been caused by various levels of imprecise HLA typings of recipients and their graft donors, small sample sizes and/or multiple heterogeneity factors, i.e. ethnicity of recipients and donors, centers, surgeons, transplant experience, post-operative immunosuppression protocols, and the storage method and quality control of the corneal grafts. Consequently, there is no logical reason why we should not apply the same ethical and moral imperatives that govern other transplantations to the practice of corneal transplantation, i.e. to HLA type and match and select the most suitable donor/recipient combinations and thus provide patients with corneal grafts with a high probability of good long-term function.

We should consider the nominal cost of HLA typing and matching as clearly secondary to the cost of maintaining the quality of life of corneal transplant recipients and the prevention of the psychological trauma of graft rejection. HLA typing and matching is clearly more cost-effective than retransplantation. Reductions in the number of retransplants inevitably lead to a better utilization of the still inadequate number of available corneal graft donors and a reduction in the number of patients waiting for a transplant.

Acknowledgments

Supported in part by the Dutch Cornea Foundation, the Eurotransplant Foundation, J.A. Cohen Institute IRS, and the Dutch National Reference Center for Histocompatibility. The Bio Implant Services (BIS) Foundation was responsible for the logistical aspects involved in the collection of the donor corneas, their transportation to the storage and control facility in Amsterdam, matching of donors and recipients and the final delivery of the donor corneas to the transplantation centers. We also wish to acknowledge the contribution by numerous donor centers for the corneal grafts used in this study.

References

1   Gibson T, Medawar PB: The fate of skin homografts in man. J Anat (Lond) 1943;77:299.
2   Medawar PB: Immunity to homologous grafted skin. II. The relationship between the antigens of blood and skin. Br J Exp Pathol 1946;27:15.
3   Van Rood JJ: Leukocyte grouping. A method and its application; thesis, Leiden 1962.
4   Frelinger JA, Shreffler DC: The major histocompatibility complexes; in: Benacerraf B (ed): Immunogenetics and Immunodeficiency Lancaster, MTP, 1975.
5   Völker-Dieben HJ, D'Amaro J, de Lange P: Interaction between prognostic factors for corneal allograft survival. Transplant Proc 1989;21:3135.
6   Irschick E, Miller K, Berger M: Studies on the mechanism of tolerance induced by short-term immunosuppression with cyclosporine in high-risk corneal allograft recipients. I. Analysis of CTL precursor frequencies. Transplantation 1989;48:986–992.
7   Rowden G: The Langerhans cell. Crit Rev Immunol 1981;2:95–180.
8   Pepose JS, Gardner KM, Nestor MS, Foos RY, Pettit TH: Detection of HLA class I and II antigens in rejected human corneal allografts. Ophthalmology 1985;92:1480–1484.
9   Ardjomand N, Komericki P, Radner H, Algner R, Reich ME: Corneal Langerhans cells. Behavior during storage in organ culture. Ophthalmology 1997;94:703–706.
10   Niederkorn JY, Ross JR, He Y: Effect of donor Langerhans cells on corneal graft rejection. J Invest Dermatol 1992;99:104S–106S.
11   Treseler PA, Sanfilippo F: Relative contribution of major histocompatibility complex antigens to the immunogenicity of corneal allografts. Transplantation 1986;41:508–514.
12   Claas FHJ, Roelen DL, D'Amaro J, Völker-Dieben HJ: The role of HLA in corneal transplantation; in Immunology of Corneal Transplantation. Buren/NL, Aeolus Press, 1994, p 47.
13   Allansmith MR, Fine M, Payne R: Histocompatibility typing and corneal transplantation. Trans Am Acad Ophthalmol Otol 1974;78:445.
14   Ducrey NM, Glauser MP, Frei PC: Corneal transplantation: ABO blood groups and HLA compatibility. Ann Ophthalmol 1980(July):880.

15   The Collaborative Corneal Transplantation Studies (CCTS) Research Group: Effectiveness of histocompatibility matching in high-risk corneal transplantation. Arch Ophthalmol 1992;110: 1392.

16   Gore SM, Vail A, Bradley BA, Rogers CA, Easty DL, Armitage WJ: HLA-DR matching in corneal transplantation. Systematic review of published data. Transplantation 1995;60:1033.

17   Bradley BA, Gore SM, Rogers CA, Armitage WJ, Easty DL: Negative effect of HLA-DR matching on corneal rejection. Transplant Proc 1995;27:1392.

18   Vail A, Gore SM, Bradley BA, Easty Dl, Rogers CA, Armitage WJ: Conclusions of the corneal transplant follow-up study. Br J Ophthalmol 1997;81:631.

19   Batchelor JR, Casey TA, Gibbs DC, Lloyd DF, Werb A, Prasad SS, James A: HLA matching and corneal grafting. Lancet 1976;i:551.

20   Ehlers N, Kissmeyer-Nielsen F: Influence of histocompatibility antigens on the fate of the corneal transplant; in Porter R, Knight J (eds): Corneal Graft Failure. Ciba Found Symp 15. Amsterdam, Associated Scientific Publishers, 1973, p 307.

21   Sanfilippo F, MacQueen JM, Vaughn WK, Foulks GN: Reduced graft rejection with good HLA-A and -B matching in high-risk corneal transplantation. N Engl J Med 1986;315:29.

22   Völker-Dieben HJ, D'Amaro J, Kok-van Alphen CC: Hierarchy of prognostic factors for corneal allograft survival. Aust NZ J Ophthalmol 1987;15:11.

23   Völker-Dieben HJ, D'Amaro J: Corneal transplantation: A single-center experience 1976–1988; in Terasaki P (ed): Clinical Transplants 1988. Los Angeles, UCLA Tissue Typing Laboratory, 1988, chapt 27, p 249.

24   Völker-Dieben HJ, D'Amaro J, Kruit PJ, de Lange P: Interaction between prognostic factors for corneal allograft survival. Transplant Proc 1989;21:3135.

25   D'Amaro J, Völker-Dieben HJ, Kruit PJ, de Lange P, Schipper R: Influence of pretransplant sensitization on the survival of corneal allografts. Transplant Proc 1991;23:368.

26   Roy R, Wagner E, Boisjoly HM: Role of lymphocytotoxic antibodies in human corneal graft rejection; in Tsuji K, Aizawa M, Sasazuki T (eds): HLA 1991. Proc 11th Histocompatibility Workshop and Conference. Oxford, Oxford University Press, 1991, vol 2, p 480.

27   Boisjoly HM, Tourigny R, Bazin R, Loughrea PA, Dube I, Chamberland G, Berier J, Roy R: Risk factors of corneal graft failure. Ophthalmology 1993;100:1728.

28   Hoffmann F, Tregel M, Noske W, Bunte S: HLA-B and -DR match reduces the allograft reaction after keratoplasty. Ger J Ophthalmol 1994;3:110.

29   Taylor CJ, Dyer PA: Histocompatibility antigens. Eye 1995;9:173.

30   Van Rood JJ, Claas FHJ, Doxiadis IIN, Schreuder GMT, Persijn GG: Current opinions: HLA typing; in Terasaki P (ed): Clinical Transplants 1993. Los Angeles, UCLA Tissue Typing Laboratory, 1993, pp 434–435.

31   Penn I: Occurrence of cancers in immunosuppressed organ transplant recipients; in Terasaki P, Cecka M (eds): Clinical Transplants 1994. Los Angeles, UCLA Tissue Typing Laboratory, 1994, pp 99–109.

32   Kinlen LJ, Sheil AGR, Peto J, Doll R: Collaborative United Kingdom-Australasian study of cancer in patients treated with immunosuppressive drugs. Br Med J 1979;ii:1461–1466.

33   Völker-Dieben HJ, Claas FHJ, Schreuder GMT, Schipper RF, Pels E, Persijn GG, Smits J, D'Amaro J: Beneficial effect of HLA-DR matching on the survival of corneal allografts. Transplantation 2000;70:641–648.

34   Kaplan EI, Meier P: Nonparametric estimations from incomplete observations. JAMA 1958; 53:457.

35   Peto R, Pike MC, Armitage P, Breslow NE, Cox DR, Howard SV, Mantel N, McPherson K, Peto J, Smith PG: Design and analysis of randomized clinical trials requiring prolonged observation of each patient. II. Analysis and examples. Br J Cancer 1976;35:1.

36   Cox DR: Regression models and life tables. J R Statist Soc B 1972;34:187–220.

37   Schreuder GMT: HLA typing by alloantibodies and monoclonal antibodies; in Bidwell JL, Navarrete C (eds): Histocompatibility Testing. London, Imperial College Press, 2001, pp 49–64.

38   Schipper RF, D'Amaro J: Population genetics of the human major histocompatibility complex; in Bidwell JL, Navarrete C (eds): Histocompatibility Testing. London, Imperial College Press, 2001, pp 395–416.

39 Verduyn W, Doxiadis IIN, Anholts J, Drabbels JJM, Naipal A, D'Amaro J, Persijn GG, Giphary MJ, Schreuder GMT: Biotinylated DRB sequence-specific oligonucleotides. Comparison to serologic HLA-DR typing of organ donors in Eurotransplant. Hum Immunol 1993;37:59–67.

40 Cohen B, Persijn G, De Meester J (eds): Eurotransplant Annual Report, 1997, p 49.

41 Hardy GH: Mendelian proportions in a mixed population. Science 1908;28:49–50.

42 Weinberg W: On the demonstration of heredity in man; in Boyer SH (ed): Papers on Human Genetics 1908. Englewood Cliffs, Prentice-Hall, 1963.

43 Boisjoly HM, Roy R, Dube I, Laughrea PA, Michaud R, Douville P, Heebert J: HLA-A, -B and -DR matching in corneal transplantation. Ophthalmology 1986;93:1290–1297.

44 Hopkins KA, Maguire MG, Fink NE, Bias WB: Reproducibility of HLA-A, -B and -DR typing using peripheral blood samples: Results of retyping in the CCTS. Hum Immunol 1992;33:132.

45 Gjertson DW: Update: Center effects; in Terasaki P (ed): Clinical Transplants 1990. Los Angeles, UCLA Tissue Typing Laboratory, 1990, pp 375–383.

46 Bodmer JG, Rocques P, Bodmer WF, Colombani J, Degos J, Dausset J: Joint report of the 5th International Histocompatibility Workshop; in Dausset J, Colombani J (eds): Histocompatibility Testing 1972. Munksgaard, Copenhagen, 1972, pp 619–648.

47 Batchelor JR, Morris PJ, Walford RL, Dumble L, Law W, Kirk R, Case J: Studies on HL-A in a Fijian population; in Dausset J, Colombani J (eds): Histocompatibility Testing 1972. Munksgaard, Copenhagen, 1972, p 283.

48 Goulmy E: Human minor histocompatibility antigens. Curr Opin Immunol 1996;8:75–81.

49 Goulmy E, Pool J, Van Loghem E, Völker-Dieben HJ: The role of human minor histocompatibility antigens in graft failure. A mini review. Eye 1995;9:180–184.

50 Streilein JW: Anterior chamber associated immune deviation: The privilege of immunity in the eye. Surv Ophthalmol 1990;35:67–73.

51 Liew FY: Regulation of delayed-type hypersensitivity. VI. Antigen-specific suppressor T cells and suppressor factor for delayed-type hypersensitivity to histocompatibility antigens. Transplantation 1982;33:69–76.

52 Niederkorn JY: The immunology of corneal transplantation; in Immuno-Ophthalmology. Dev Opthalmol. Basel, Karger, 1999, vol 30, pp 129–140.

53 Jager MJ: Corneal Langerhans cells and ocular immunology. Reg Immunol 1992;4:186–195.

54 Roelen RL, Datema G, Van Bree S, Zhang L, Van Rood JJ, Claas FHJ: Evidence that antibody formation against a certain HLA alloantigen is associated not with a quantitative but with a qualitative change in the cytotoxic T cells recognizing the same antigen. Transplantation 1992;53: 899–903.

55 Foets BJ, van den Oord JJ, Billiau A, Van Damme J, Missotten L: Heterogeneous induction of major histocompatibility complex class II antigens on corneal endothelium by interferon-γ. Invest Ophthalmol Vis Sci 1991;32:341.

56 Iwata M, Kiritoshi A, Roat MI, Yagihashi A, Thoft RA: Regulation of HLA class II antigen expression on cultured corneal epithelium by interferon-γ. Invest Ophthalmol Vis Sci 1992;33:2714.

Prof. Dr. H.J. Völker-Dieben
PO Box 7057
1007 MB Amsterdam (The Netherlands)
Tel. +31 20 4444795, Fax +31 20 4444745, E-Mail HJM.Voelker-Dieben@VUMC.NL

Sundmacher R (ed): Adequate HLA Matching in Keratoplasty.
Dev Ophthalmol. Basel, Karger, 2003, vol 36, pp 42–49

....

HLA Class I and II Matching Improves Prognosis in Penetrating Normal-Risk Keratoplasty

Thomas Reinhard[a], Daniel Böhringer[a], Jürgen Enczmann[b],
Gesine Kögler[b], Susanne Mayweg[a], Peter Wernet[b], Rainer Sundmacher[a]

[a]Eye Hospital and Lions Cornea Bank North Rhine-Westphalia and [b]Institute for Transplantation Immunology and Cell Therapeutics, Molecular Genetic Laboratory, Heinrich-Heine University, Düsseldorf, Germany

Abstract

Background: HLA matching in penetrating keratoplasty is still neglected in most eye clinics. This is due to contradictory results of studies performed in the past. Different surgical techniques in multicenter studies, missing risk differentiation in high-risk situations and faulty HLA typing can be identified as the main reasons for these contradictory results. In this monocenter study, the value of HLA class I and II matching (A, B, DR loci) was examined in a homogenous group of 398 normal-risk keratoplasty patients using modern typing techniques.

Methods: Penetrating normal-risk keratoplasty was performed in two groups of patients (group I with 0–2, group II with 3–6 mismatches in the A/B/DR loci). Surgery was done by 3 experienced surgeons according to a standardized scheme. Also, postoperative therapy and controls were standardized. There were no statistically significant differences between the two study groups as regards number of AB0 or H-Y compatibilities, patient age, patient gender, ratio of previous intraocular surgery, ratio of triple procedures, indication for surgery, follow-up period, donor age, donor gender, post-mortem time of the graft and endothelial cell density of the graft at the end of organ culture. HLA typing was performed in a quality-controlled laboratory, serologically for HLA class I (A and B loci) and moleculargenetically for HLA class II (DR locus).

Results: Four years postoperatively, the ratio of clear and rejection-free graft survival was 91% in group I and 67% in group II (Kaplan-Meier estimation, log rank test, p = 0.03). Monovariate analysis in the Cox model gave no influence of solitary HLA class I *or* II matching, but only an influence of combined HLA class I *and* II matching (p = 0.03).

Conclusions: In this monocenter study with proper typing techniques the beneficial effect of HLA class I *plus* II matching on clear and rejection-free graft survival could be demonstrated in a homogenous group of normal-risk keratoplasty patients.

Background

In this study, faults committed in previous studies as enumerated in the Introduction of this book were avoided by a monocenter design with only 3 experienced cornea surgeons, by choosing normal-risk keratoplasty patients as participants, thus excluding non-immunological reasons for graft failure, and by performing HLA typing in an optimally quality-controlled laboratory, serologically for class I and moleculargenetically for class II.

Patients and Methods

Penetrating normal-risk keratoplasty was performed in a homogenous monocenter group of 398 patients after obtaining written informed consent from every patient.

Patient Selection

Only patients undergoing first keratoplasty within an avascular host cornea were included. All grafts with a diameter of 7.7 mm were positioned centrally. Indications for surgery were keratoconus, Fuchs' endothelial dystrophy, bullous keratopathy and non-herpetic, avascular scars. None of the patients had a history of severe surface disorders, glaucoma or herpetic eye disease.

Since 1995, HLA typing has been performed in all normal-risk keratoplasty patients attending the clinic. All patients were placed on a waiting list for a maximum of 6 months. If a graft with 0–2 mismatches (group I) on the HLA A, B and DR loci had not been found within this period, a graft with 3–6 mismatches was assigned (group II). Group I comprised 65 patients, group II 333 patients: 1 patient received a graft with 0, 28 with 1, 36 with 2, 69 with 3, 114 with 4, 106 with 5 and 44 with 6 mismatches. Patient, donor, graft and surgery data of both study groups are enumerated in table 1a and b.

HLA Typing and Matching

All serologic HLA A, B and all molecular genetic HLA DRB, DRQB typings of donors and recipients were performed in a single laboratory accredited by the American Society for Histocompatibility and Immunogenetics [1]. For HLA matching only broad antigens (class I: A, B; class II: DR) were considered.

Distribution of Blood Group Mismatches (AB0)

AB0 typing was performed serologically in the same optimally quality-controlled laboratory. In group I 39/65 patients and in group II 178/333 patients received AB0-matched grafts (donor A/recipient A or AB, donor B/recipient B or AB, donor AB/recipient AB, donor 0/recipient A, B, AB or 0) (χ^2 test, p = 0.6).

Table 1. Patient data (***a***) and donor and graft data (***b***) of the study

	0–2 mismatches	3–6 mismatches	p
a. *Patient data*			
Age, years[1]	53.7 ± 21.6	59.2 ± 19.6	n.s.
Gender, f/m[2]	41/24	173/160	n.s.
Previous i.o. surgery[1]	24.9%	28.3%	n.s.
Triple/pkp[2]	15.2%	20.2%	n.s.
Indication for surgery, kc/Fed/other[2]	22/21/22	102/116/115	n.s.
Follow-up, days[1]	582 ± 419	613 ± 463	n.s.
b. *Donor and graft data*			
Age, years[1]	61.1 ± 18.4	60.3 ± 17.3	n.s.
Gender, f/m[2]	32/33	123/210	n.s.
Post-mortem time, h[1]	9.4 ± 10.1	13.4 ± 14.9	n.s.
Storage time in organ culture, days[1]	17.3 ± 4.3	15.4 ± 4.6	0.03
Ecd directly after organ culture, cells/mm² [1]	2,363 ± 263	2,311 ± 252	n.s.

[1]ANOVA, χ^2 test.

n.s. = not significant; kk = keratoconus; Fed = Fuchs endothelial dystrophy; other = bullous keratopathy or non-herpetic avascular scars; Ecd = endothelial cell density.

Distribution of Minor Histocompatibility H-Y Mismatches

In group I 46/65 patients and in group II 238/333 patients received H-Y-matched grafts (donor male/recipient male, donor female/recipient male or female) (χ^2 test, p = 0.4).

Grafts

All grafts were preserved in organ culture according to the guidelines of the European Eye Bank Association [2]. Preoperative evaluation of the graft endothelium was performed in hypotonic solution under the phase-contrast microscope the day before penetrating keratoplasty [3]. This examination was proven to deliver reproducible results [4].

Penetrating Keratoplasty, Postoperative Treatment and Controls

Surgery was done by 3 experienced surgeons in retrobulbar anesthesia according to a standardized scheme. Modified Franceschetti trephines with the diameters of 7.5 mm (recipient) and 7.7 mm (donor) were used. Graft fixation was performed with a double running cross-stitch suture with Nylon 10.0 [5]. If necessary, cataract surgery was done simultaneously (table 1a). After surgery, gentamycin ointment was administered at least until the graft was covered with a complete epithelial layer. Then corticosteroid eyedrops (prednisolone-21-acetate 1%) were given 5 times daily and tapered during the first 5 postoperative months. Systemic corticosteroids were administered for only 3 weeks postoperatively. Acetazolamide was administered in a daily dose of 500 mg for 5 days postoperatively. Controls of the graft at the slitlamp were scheduled 6 weeks, 4, 12 and 18 months postoperatively and thereafter annually.

Immune Reactions

Endothelial immune reactions were diagnosed via endothelial precipitates and stromal edema, stromal immune reactions via nummular infiltrates without preceding infectious (adenoviral) background [6]. All patients received corticosteroid eyedrops (prednisolone-21-acetate 1%) every hour until elimination of all precipitates. Furthermore, a subconjunctival injection with betamethasone-21-acetate was performed. Topical corticosteroids were tapered individually. In severe cases, systemic corticosteroids at a daily oral dose of 1 mg fluocortolone/kg body mass were administered additionally and tapered within 3 weeks.

Statistical Analysis

All statistical evaluation was performed using SPSS Windows NT 4.0 (Microsoft Corp., Redmond, Calif., USA). Clear graft survival, ratio of grafts without immune reactions and rejection-free graft survival were calculated according to Kaplan and Meier [7]. All Kaplan-Meier curves were compared via log rank test. Monovariate analysis was performed by entering patient, donor, graft and surgery data into the Cox model.

Results

Four years postoperatively, clear graft survival in group I was 100% and in group II 83% ($p = 0.065$), ratio of rejection-free grafts 91% in group I and 73% in group II ($p = 0.049$) and ratio of clear and rejection-free graft survival 91% in group I and 67% in group II ($p = 0.03$) (fig. 1a–c).

Reasons for graft failure in group II were irreversible immune reactions in 8 patients and chronic endothelial cell loss in 3 patients. In group I, 4 immune reactions were recorded. All were reversible. In group II, 50 of 58 immune reactions were reversible.

Monovariate analysis in the Cox model gave no influence of solitary HLA class I or II matching ($p = 0.31$ and $p = 0.13$, respectively), but only an influence of combined HLA class I and II matching ($p = 0.03$) on clear and rejection-free graft survival.

Discussion

Many studies were performed within the past three decades considering the effects of HLA matching in penetrating keratoplasty. They delivered contradictory results [8–21]. In this study the beneficial effect of HLA class I plus II matching on clear and rejection-free graft survival after penetrating normal-risk keratoplasty could be demonstrated. The main difference between the two study groups was the

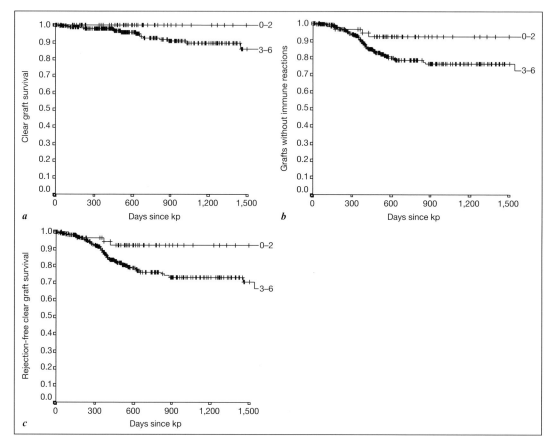

Fig. 1. HLA matching in 398 normal-risk penetrating keratoplasties (kp): (*a*) clear graft survival (0–2/3–6 mismatches, log rank test: p = 0.065); (*b*) grafts without immune reactions (0–2/3–6 mismatches, log rank test: p = 0.049) and (*c*) rejection-free clear graft survival (0–2/3–6 mismatches, log rank test: p = 0.03).

number of HLA mismatches. All other factors possibly influencing study outcome were comparable. Compared to other studies, this study offers five advantages:

(1) In a monocenter design only 3 experienced surgeons performed all transplantations according to a standardized scheme. Also, all postoperative therapy and all postoperative examinations were performed in a standardized manner.

(2) Only normal-risk keratoplasty patients were considered for the study in order to minimize the influence of non-immunological risk factors.

(3) Various patient, donor and graft parameters may influence clear and rejection-free graft survival. In this study, patient age, patient gender, ratio of previous intraocular surgery, ratio of triple procedures, indication for surgery and

follow-up did not show statistically significant differences between the two study groups. The same is true for donor age, donor gender, post-mortem time and endothelial cell density of the graft at the end of standardized organ culture. Only storage time in organ culture was statistically significantly longer in group I. If this had an influence on the study results one might expect worse results in the group with the longer storage period [22, 23]. The contrary, however, was observed.

(4) In the past, the influence of blood group compatibility on graft prognosis was discussed controversially [18]. It may be important, therefore, that the number of patients with blood group compatibilities was comparable in both study groups. An influence of minor histocompatibility mismatches on graft prognosis was found by Streilein [24] in the mouse penetrating keratoplasty model. The only minor histocompatibility antigen investigated in this study was H-Y. In the two study groups the ratio of patients with minor histocompatibility antigen H-Y mismatches was similar.

(5) All HLA typing was performed in only one quality-controlled laboratory, serologically for class I and moleculargenetically for class II. In the past, serological typing of class I was shown to deliver reliable results [31]. This is not the case for HLA class II, even if material from heart-beating donors is analyzed [25, 26]. In penetrating keratoplasty, however, blood from cornea donors is often obtained up to 72 h after death. In this study, therefore, the DR locus was determined exclusively by moleculargenetic means [1].

The expression of class I and II antigens in the cornea is still controversially discussed. Streilein [27] identified reduced expression of MHC antigens as one reason for the immune privilege of corneal grafts. Newsome et al. [28] demonstrated the presence of class I antigens on epithelial, stromal and endothelial corneal cells. In contrast, class II antigens are regularly expressed only on epithelial Langerhans' cells [29]. After incubation with interferon-γ, however, class II antigens are expressed on all corneal cells including the endothelium [30, 31]. CD4 T cells are the main source of interferon-γ [32]. In the rat-penetrating keratoplasty model, CD4 T cells were found even in syngeneic grafts [32]. Possibly, an elevation of interferon-γ levels in the graft may already be caused by a surgical trauma such as penetrating (normal-risk) keratoplasty.

The evolution in keratoplasty has been such that the early attempts to exploit the theoretical advantages of HLA matching had unavoidably too often been technically weak so that the probability of negative or questionable results was high. On the other hand, the introduction of more and more efficient systemic immunodrugs has brought about such a quick and important breakthrough in the prognosis especially of high-risk keratoplasties that the current 'neglect' of the HLA system is understandable from this experience.

We have shown that even patients with a normal-risk keratoplasty benefit from a good HLA A/B plus HLA DR match. As others [26, 33] have recently published that HLA matching is beneficial also in high-risk and in mixed-risk groups, these unison our reports mean that HLA matching must now be regarded as basically beneficial for all keratoplasty patients.

It does not follow that HLA matching must actually be required for every patient. For the time being the practical consequences will anyway be limited because the logistics for a widespread application of matching principles in keratoplasty do simply not yet exist in most parts of the world. It must be discussed, however, whether it will be worthwhile to establish such logistics. We vigorously favor such a project.

For normal-risk patients we would expect that their transplants' life span, which currently on an average is not longer than about 10–20 years, will be considerably expanded. This is extremely important for all patients under the age of about 60. For high-risk patients, efficient HLA matching will help to bring about conditions in which tolerance of the graft by the host is established more easily and more efficiently and longer lasting than with systemic immunomodulative drugs alone. The application of the latter is often limited by severe side effects or their effect may be insufficient when given as the only measure.

Thus, all keratoplasty patients should benefit to various degrees from HLA matching, and it is our hope that this paper together with those of others [26, 33] will lead to a re-evaluation and reappraisal of HLA matching in keratoplasty.

Acknowledgement

Supported by Bio Implant Services, Leiden, The Netherlands.

References

1   Wernet P, Kögler G, Enczmann J, Kuhröber A, Knipper A, Bonte W, Reinhard T, Sundmacher R: Rapid method for successful HLA class I and II typing from cadaveric blood for direct matching in cornea transplantation. Graefes Arch Clin Exp Ophthalmol 1998;236:507–512.
2   Pels L, Maas H, Tullo A: European Eye Bank Association Directory, ed 8, 2000.
3   Böhnke M: Spendergewebe für die Keratoplastik. Klin Monatsbl Augenheilkd 1991;198:563–571.
4   Reinhard T, Holzwarth D, Spelsberg H, Dahmen N, Sundmacher R: Wissensbasierte Bildanalyse von Hornhauttransplantaten. Klin Monatsbl Augenheilkd 1999;214:407–411.
5   Hoffmann F: Nahttechnik bei perforierender Keratoplastik. Klin Monatsbl Augenheilkd 1976; 169:584–590.
6   Allredge OC, Krachmer JH: Clinical types of corneal transplant reaction. Arch Ophthalmol 1981; 99:599–604.
7   Kaplan EL, Meier P: Nonparametric estimation from incomplete observations. J Am Stat Assoc 1958;53:457–481.
8   Gibbs DC, Batchelor R, Werb A, Schlesinger W, Casey TA: The influence of tissue-type compatibility on the fate of full-thickness corneal grafts. Trans Ophthalmol Soc 1974;94:101–126.
9   Vannas S: Histocompatibility in corneal grafting. Invest Ophthalmol 1975;14:883–886.
10 Stark WJ, Hugh RT, Bias WB, Maumenee AE: Histocompatibility (HLA) antigens and keratoplasty. Am J Ophthalmol 86:595–604.

11 Ehlers N, Kissmeyer-Nielsen F: Corneal transplantation and HLA histocompatibility. Acta Ophthalmol 1979;57:738–741.

12 Foulks GN, Sanfilippo FP, Locasio JA, MacQueen JM, Dawson DV: Histocompatibility testing for keratoplasty in high-risk patients. Ophthalmology 1983;90:239–244.

13 Sanfilippo F, MacQueen JM, Vaughn WK, Foulks GN: Reduced graft rejection with good HLA-A and -B matching in high-risk corneal transplantation. N Engl J Med 1986;315:29–35.

14 Völker-Dieben HJ, D'Amaro J, Kruit PJ, Lange P: Interaction between prognostic factors for corneal allograft survival. Transplant Proc 1989;21:3135–3138.

15 Boisjoly HM, Roy R, Bernard PM, Dubé I, Laughrea PA, Bazin R: Association between corneal allograft reactions and HLA compatibility. Ophthalmology 1990;97:1689–1698.

16 Baggesen K, Ehlers N, Lamm LU: HLA-DR/RFLP compatible corneal grafts. Acta Ophthalmol 1991;69:229–233.

17 Beekhuis WH, van Rij G, Renardel de Lavalette JG, Rinkel-van Driel E, Persijn G, D'Amaro J: Corneal graft survival in HLA-A- and HLA-B-matched transplantations in high-risk cases with retrospective review of HLA-DR compatibility. Cornea 1991;10:9–12.

18 CCTS: Effectiveness of histocompatibility matching in high-risk corneal transplantation. Arch Ophthalmol 1992;110:1392–1403.

19 Vail A, Gore SM, Bradley BA, Easty DL, Rogers CA, Armitage WJ: Conclusions of the corneal transplant follow-up study. Br J Ophthalmol 1997;81:631–636.

20 Hoffmann F, Pahlitzsch T: Predisposing factors in corneal graft rejection. Cornea 1989;8:215–219.

21 Hoffmann F, Tregel M, Noske W, Bünte S: HLA-B and -DR match reduces the allograft rejection after keratoplasty. Ger J Ophthalmol 1994;3:100–104.

22 Armitage WJ, Easty DL: Factors influencing the suitability of organ-cultured corneas for transplantation. Invest Ophthalmol Vis Sci 1997;38:16–24.

23 Borderie VM, Scheer S, Touzeau O: Donor organ cultured corneal tissue selection before penetrating keratoplasty. Br J Ophthalmol 1998;82:382–388.

24 Streilein JW: Immunobiology and immunopathology of corneal transplantation; in Streilein JW (ed): Immune Response and the Eye. Chem Immunol. Basel, Karger, 1999, vol 79, pp 186–206.

25 Hopkins KA, Maguire MG, Fink NE, Bias WB: Reproducibility of HLA-A, -B, and -DR typing using peripheral blood samples: Results of retyping in the CCTS. Hum Immunol 1992;22:132.

26 Völker-Dieben HJ, Claas FHJ, Schreuder GMT, Schipper RF, Pels E, Persijn GG, Smits J, D'Amaro J: Beneficial effect of HLA-DR matching on the survival of corneal allografts. Transplantation 2000;70:640–648.

27 Streilein J: Unraveling immune privilege. Science 1995;270:1158–1159.

28 Newsome DA, Takasugi M, Kenyon K, Stark WF, Opelz G: Human corneal cells in vitro: Morphology and histocompatibility antigens of pure cell populations. Invest Ophthalmol Vis Sci 1974;13:23–32.

29 Jager M: Corneal Langerhans cells and ocular immunology. Reg Immunol 1992;4:186–195.

30 Donelly JJ, Li W, Rockey JH, Prendergast RA: Induction of class II alloantigen expression on corneal endothelium in vivo and in vitro. Invest Ophthalmol Vis Sci 185;26:575–580.

31 Young E, Stark WJ, Prendergast RA: Immunology of corneal allograft rejection: HLA-DR antigens on human corneal cells. Invest Ophthalmol Vis Sci 1985;26:571–574.

32 Vilcek J, Jumming L: Interferon-γ; in Delves PJ, Roitt IM (ed): Encyclopedia of Immunology. San Diego, Academic Press, 1999, pp 1421–1426.

33 Beekhuis WH: Langzeitergebnisse bei HLA-A- und B-gematchter Hochrisiko-Keratoplastik. Ophthalmologe 2001;98:S6–S7.

Thomas Reinhard, MD
Eye Hospital and Lions Cornea Bank North Rhine-Westphalia,
Heinrich-Heine University, D–40225 Düsseldorf (Germany)
Tel. +49 211 8118795, Fax +49 211 8118796, E-Mail thomas.reinhard@uni-duesseldorf.de

Sundmacher R (ed): Adequate HLA Matching in Keratoplasty.
Dev Ophthalmol. Basel, Karger, 2003, vol 36, pp 50–55

....

Individual Analysis of Expected Time on the Waiting List for HLA-Matched Corneal Grafts

D. Böhringer[a], T. Reinhard[a], J. Enczmann[b], E. Godehard[c],
R. Sundmacher[a]

[a]Eye Hospital and Lions Cornea Bank North Rhine-Westphalia; [b]Institute for
Transplantation Immunology, and [c]Clinic of Cardiac and Thoracic Surgery,
University Hospital Heinrich Heine University, Düsseldorf, Germany

Abstract

Objective: Recent studies report the beneficial effect of HLA matching for long-term
prognosis of penetrating keratoplasty (kp). This improvement of prognosis, however, has to
be weighed against the additional time on the waiting list due to the search for a HLA-
compatible graft. Reliable estimation of this additional waiting period is a prerequisite for
informed consent on the waiting policy.

Methods: A mathematical model based on survival analysis and HLA haplotype
frequencies was used to estimate time on the waiting list for each of 1,400 HLA-typed
patients registered at the Lions Cornea Bank NRW. Additionally, the waiting period of each
patient was retrospectively determined. Both values were tested for correlation. This analysis was performed for acceptance of up to two mismatches on HLA-A, -B and -DR.

Results: When accepting two, one and zero mismatches, median predicted waiting
period was 1 ± 6, 7 ± 49 and 17 ± 159 months respectively. Median waiting period in
retrospective simulation was 1 ± 3, 5 ± 9 and 15 ± 14 months. Correlation of values from
the predictive formula and simulation was statistically significant ($p < 0.0001$).

Conclusion: Predicted time on the waiting list is a valuable tool for management of
HLA matching in kp.

Background

Unlike in bone marrow and kidney transplantation, HLA matching in
keratoplasty (kp) is currently considered optional. This is due to ACAID [1, 2]

in normal-risk kp and to availability of optimized systemic immunosuppressive regimens in high-risk cases [3]. Recent evidence [4], however, suggests that prognosis in low-risk as well as in high-risk kp can be further improved by HLA class I and II matching. Naturally, any improvement of prognosis has to be weighed against time on the waiting list due to search for an HLA-compatible graft. This waiting period may be associated with social costs of blindness [5] and more often with social costs of reduced working ability as well as with severe reductions in quality of life. Waiting for much longer than 1 year for many individuals is hard to accept. Thus, when a long waiting period has to be considered likely, a randomly assigned graft with appropriate potent immuno-suppression may often be preferable for a patient for different and often individual reasons. This is especially true, of course, in normal-risk kp, *where mid-term prognosis* is already excellent [6, 7] and supportive HLA matching for most patients will not so much improve their medium-term prognosis than their long-term prognosis. A reliable method for predicting the waiting period is thus necessary for informed consent on the waiting policy, and the pros and cons have to be discussed with every patient individually.

A method for predicting waiting periods with respect to HLA compatibility is derived from definition of HLA-compatible grafts and their HLA frequencies. It is consecutively validated by means of simulation.

Methods

Frequency of HLA-Compatible Grafts

For any recipient, the frequency of HLA-compatible donors (*matchability score* [8]) can either be determined empirically by means of simulation [9], or derived analytically. Only the analytical approach yields robust and reproducible individual matchability scores and is thus defined in the following.

$3^{(n-m)}$ different HLA totally compatible donor genotypes exist for each recipient (n is the count of HLA loci considered and m the count of homozygous loci of the individual). This number increases as more loci are considered, but the total number of genotypes increases faster, so that the more loci are considered, the lower is the proportion of compatible donors. Commonly, three HLA loci (A, B and DR) are considered, so for each recipient completely heterozygous at the loci considered, 27 different compatible genotypes (donors) are to be considered.

The total percentage of the donor population matching a specific HLA genotype (recipient) is well approximated by the sum of the individual frequencies of all HLA-compatible diplotypes. These diplotypes each comprise two haplotypes bearing only as much alleles foreign to the recipient (commonly zero) as considered acceptable by the clinician.

When only the HLA loci A, B and DR are considered, individual haplotype frequencies can be retrieved from databases of three locus haplotype frequencies for the respective donor population [10]. In this investigation, a database of the 1,516 most common three locus HLA haplotype frequencies in the German population [www.BMDW.org] was used for calculation. Only broad alleles were considered. Only haplotypes of a frequency greater than 0.03% were addressed.

The frequency of any HLA genotype is the sum of the products of all haplotype frequencies of haplotypes bearing the respective alleles (Mendelian segregation of HLA alleles). When one mismatch is accepted, appropriate frequencies from three locus haplotype frequencies are combined with appropriate two locus haplotype frequencies (canonically derived from three locus haplotype frequencies). When two mismatches are accepted, only the appropriate two locus haplotype frequencies are considered.

Estimation of the Waiting Period

The rate of HLA-compatible grafts available per day equals the product of the daily rate of new HLA-typed grafts and the total frequency of HLA-compatible donors. When assuming Poissonian distribution of donors, the expected waiting period is reciprocal to the daily rate of new HLA-compatible grafts. This relationship is based on survival analysis: the rate of HLA-compatible grafts can be interpreted as a death rate and each HLA-compatible transplantation can be thought of as an event of death. Expected lifespan, the reciprocal of death rate, then obviously equals the waiting period. This formula is summarized in equation 1.

$$t = \frac{1/365}{GR \Sigma GF} \tag{1}$$

t: expected waiting period (years); *GF*: individual HLA gene frequencies of compatible diplotypes; *GR*: daily rate of new corneas for which the HLA-A, -B and -DR type is known.

Due to quality control of grafts for stringent criteria [11] and technical problems in post-mortem HLA typing, not every donor available may contribute to the matching pool. The percentage of matchable grafts is well known for all registered European cornea banks [11] and can be accounted for by including a corrective factor in the prediction algorithm.

Validation

The above model derived from survival analysis can only be considered appropriate if model predictions are significantly correlated with real waiting periods. This correlation has thus to be assessed first. Real-world waiting periods depend on multiple factors other than HLA compatibility, such as missing a compatible graft due to poor general health at scheduled transplantation. A more robust substitute for the historical real-world waiting period is the time interval from being put on the waiting list to the earliest ascertainment of an HLA-compatible graft (donor's date of death) when only donors deceased after entrance on list are considered and real-world sequence of past donors is maintained. This simulation is an estimation of the time interval each patient would have been waiting in the past if HLA compatibility had been the only criterion in past allocation. The above time interval was simulated for each of the 1,400 patients with complete HLA class I and II type (A, B and DR loci) registered at the LIONS Cornea Bank NRW. Individual HLA compatibility achieved in reality was thus ignored.

Statistics

Custom software for waiting period prediction and the program that performed the retrospective HLA matching were implemented in the computer language Perl5 as described

Table 1. Median values ± SD (months) of waiting periods generated by means of retrospective simulation and by the predictive formula adopted for the Lions Cornea Bank NRW, Germany

	Zero mismatches	One mismatch	Two mismatches
Share of recipients for which a matching graft was found	29%	71%	83%
Simulated period	15 ± 14	5 ± 9	1 ± 3
Predicted period	17 ± 159	7 ± 49	1 ± 6
Correlation of simulated and predicted periods	R = 0.28 p < 0.001	R = 0.36 p < 0.001	R = 0.45 p < 0.001

The percentage of recipients for which a compatible match was found is shown. R: Correlation coefficient, p: significance of bivariate correlation. Parameters (long-term means) are: 0.87 donors per day, 80% of them with complete HLA type (A, B and DR loci).

in sections *Frequency of HLA-Compatible Grafts* and *Estimation of the Waiting Period* above. Parametrical bivariate correlation analysis was performed. All time intervals were logarithmically transformed before correlation to approximate normality.

Statistics were performed using SPSS 10 on Windows NT 4.

Results

Median time intervals from simulation are well compatible with predicted waiting periods (table 1). Median difference is below 2 months. Correlations are statistically highly significant (table 1) as well.

With each HLA mismatch accepted, the share of HLA-compatible transplantations possible rises steeply.

Discussion

A method is presented for predicting time on the waiting list with respect to a recipient's HLA type by means of calculating the percentage of HLA-compatible donors and then by deriving the expected waiting period from this portion. This analysis has been performed for acceptance of zero, one and two out of six HLA mismatches. Good predictive power of the model could be demonstrated by means of simulation (table 1).

This approach neglects 'rivalry' between recipients for compatible donors. This simplification has been proven wrong in kidney transplantation [9], where each donor routinely fits numerous recipients on multicenter waiting lists. All but one recipient have to wait for the next available compatible donor, potentially multiplying real-world waiting period. In kp, however, HLA matching has been mostly considered optional up to now. This is reflected by the fact that only 18% of all patients in this study had actually been registered on the waiting list for an HLA-compatible graft in the 4 years overseen in this study. This policy compartmentalized the waiting list and drastically reduced rivalry among recipients since those with mandatory compatibility were matched with priority. The predicted waiting periods of these special recipients should be comparable to waiting periods from simulation. This underscores the predictive power of the presented method for kp waiting lists, when priority in matching is assigned to a subset of the complete waiting list. With increasing number of recipients registered for mandatory HLA compatibility, the predictive model will underestimate the real waiting period, especially for patients with a rare phenotype (for those the formula predicts waiting times greater than e.g. 100 years). For them, a matched donor will practically not be available, whereas for other patients it is easy to find a well-matched donor. When two patients compete for the same donor, it is useful to give the graft to the patient with the rare phenotype even if the donor is better matched with the other one. This could be achieved by deriving a weighed priority score from the expected time on the waiting list, the actual time on the waiting list, and the match grade of the graft to be assigned to the competing patients.

By means of simulation as well as by prediction it has been shown that when one or two mismatches are accepted, waiting for HLA-compatible grafts is mostly achievable and thus advisable even in low-risk kp.

The method presented here is a valuable tool for managing HLA matching in kp and for discussing waiting policy on an individual basis.

Acknowledgement

Supported by Bio Implant Services Foundation, Leiden, The Netherlands.

References

1   Streilein JW: Tissue barriers, immunosuppressive microenvironments, and privileged sites: The eye's point of view. Reg Immunol 1993;5:253–268.
2   Niederkorn JY, Mellon J: Anterior chamber-associated immune deviation promotes corneal allograft survival. Invest Ophthalmol Vis Sci 1996;37:2700–2707.

3   Reinhard T, Reis A, Kutkuhn B, Voiculescu A, Sundmacher R: Mycophenolatmofetil nach
    perforierender Hochrisiko-Keratoplastik. Eine Pilotstudie. Klin Monatsbl Augenheilkd 1999;215:
    201–202.
4   Völker-Dieben HJ, Claas FH, Schreuder GM, Schipper RF, Pels E, Persijn GG, et al: Beneficial
    effect of HLA-DR matching on the survival of corneal allografts. Transplantation 2000;70:640–648.
5   Wright SE, Keeffe JE, Thies LS: Direct costs of blindness in Australia. Clin Exp Ophthalmol
    2000;28:140–142.
6   Reinhard T, Möller M, Sundmacher R: Penetrating keratoplasty in patients with atopic dermatitis
    with and without systemic cyclosporin A. Cornea 1999;18:645–651.
7   Reinhard T, Hutmacher M, Sundmacher R: Akute und chronische Immunreaktionen nach perfori-
    erender Normalrisikokeratoplastik. Klin Monatsbl Augenheilkd 1997;210:139–143.
8   Gilks WR, Gore SM, Bradley BA: Matchability in kidney transplantation. Tissue Antigens 1988;
    32:121–129.
9   Gilks WR, Gore SM, Bradley BA: Predicting match grade and waiting time to kidney transplan-
    tation. Transplantation 1991;51:618–624.
10 Schipper RF, Oudshoorn M, D'Amaro J, van der Zanden HG, de Lange P, Bakker JT, et al:
    Validation of large data sets, an essential prerequisite for data analysis: An analytical survey of the
    Bone Marrow Donors Worldwide. Tissue Antigens 1996;47:169–178.
11 Mels L, Maas H, Tullo A: European Eye Bank Association Directory. 2000:8.

Dr. med. Daniel Böhringer
Augenklinik, Postfach 101007, D–40001 Düsseldorf (Germany)
Tel. +49 211 8118795, Fax +49 211 8118796, E-Mail daniel.boehringer@uni-duesseldorf.de

Sundmacher R (ed): Adequate HLA Matching in Keratoplasty.
Dev Ophthalmol. Basel, Karger, 2003, vol 36, pp 56–61

....

Shortage in the Face of Plenty: Improving the Allocation of Corneas for Transplantation

T.M.M.H. de By

BIS Foundation, Leiden, The Netherlands

Abstract

Background: As there are plenty of potential corneal donors, theoretically there should be no shortage of corneal grafts. Practically, however, shortages have been a problem, especially with HLA-matched corneas, which are increasingly requested. This increase requires evaluation and proper adaptation to meet all requests in the future.

Methods: BIS' allocation data for corneal transplants were analyzed for the years 1998 through 2001.

Results: Allocation of matched corneas almost doubled in 2000. The waiting list for matched grafts could be reduced by one third.

Conclusions: A steep increase in demand for matched grafts could be noted by the year 2000. This signifies that the results of positive matching studies have ultimately been taken notice of by the ophthalmic surgeons with consequent adaptation of their graft orders. BIS has mostly been able to cope with these rapidly changing and increasing demands, but more efforts are continuously needed to supply those typed and matched corneas within short time. Our next step will be to offer HLA-DR matching routinely in addition to the current HLA-A/-B matching. We are looking forward with great interest to the introduction of even more specified matching algorithms in the not too far distant future, and are prepared to meet all the requirements which might be associated with such challenges.

Introduction

The quantity of HLA-typed corneas allocated by the BIS Foundation showed some remarkable changes between 1998 and 2001 [2, 3, 4–6, 7–10, 12]. These changes are influenced by technical and organizational developments.

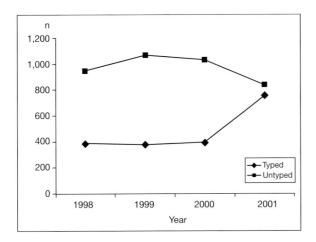

Fig. 1. Four years' allocation of available cornea grafts.

The increased scientific insight in the importance of HLA matching for nearly all patients also contributes to the observed change in allocation ratios for HLA-typed corneal grafts. Despite the upward trend in availability of HLA-typed grafts, a shortage can be observed. This shortage is expressed by the existence of a waiting list for patients in need of a well-matched graft, but also for patients who need an unmatched graft. Improved matching criteria within the BIS allocation criteria as well as timely increased donor recruitment efforts have contributed to diminish an impending shortage.

Four Years' Allocation Data

Figure 1 shows the results of allocation of HLA-typed and untyped corneas from 1998 to 2001 with a steep increase of the typed transplants by more than 90% as of the year 2000 whereas the untyped grafts decreased by some 19%. Figure 3 shows on a monthly scale this latest increase of allocated HLA-matched corneas from about 20 grafts in September 2000 to 48 grafts 1 year later. Accordingly, during this year the number of patients on the waiting list for HLA-typed corneas decreased by about one third from 333 to 230, whereas the waiting list for non-typed recipients did not show such a reduction (fig. 2).

Factors Influencing the Allocation Ratios

Four factors are responsible for the allocation ratios as observed during the period 1998 through September 2001.

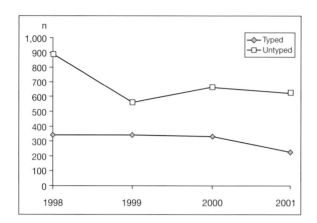

Fig. 2. Patients on the waiting list for HLA-typed corneas.

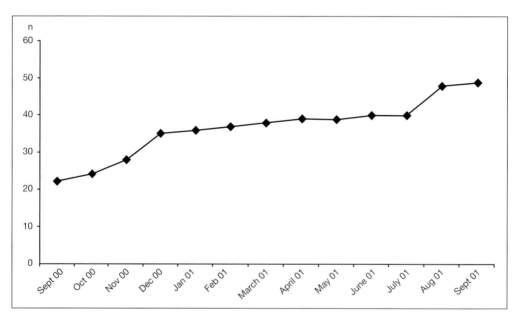

Fig. 3. Allocated HLA-typed corneas per month 2000–2001.

First, there was an increase in the number of donors for cornea donation reported to BIS in both Germany and The Netherlands, especially in the period September 2000 through August 2001. This increase was due to enforced donor recruitment activities, supported in The Netherlands by the Ministry of Health, and in Germany by individual cornea banks [1, 2]. The total number of available donors for corneal grafts in Germany, however, is still by far not enough to satisfy all demands.

Second, the allocation by BIS of HLA-typed corneal allografts in Germany has increased. This is due to the fact that the Bundesärztekammer (the responsible representatives of all German medical doctors) has issued a guideline [13] which says that typed corneas, that cannot be matched to a patient in the local waiting list of a cornea bank, shall be allocated internationally by the BIS Foundation, based upon the international allocation criteria of BIS.

Third, new DNA typing techniques have made it possible to determine the correct tissue typing despite an often poor quality of the blood sample of the deceased. The older techniques caused many undetermined laboratory results, mainly due to dead blood cells.

Fourth, the demand for DR-matched corneal grafts has increased. Although DR matching has not yet been an official allocation criterion with BIS, many physicians anticipate the introduction of matching on both HLA class I and class II antigens by BIS in the near future.

If one studies the last developments [12], different publications show that HLA matching for only class I antigens will no longer be state of the art as is convincingly presented e.g. by Völker-Dieben et al. and Reinhard et al. in this volume [10]. Furthermore, the vision of Claas [see next article] is that the clinical practice of tissue typing and HLA matching in the 21st century will not only be influenced by new and more reliable typing techniques, but also by totally new matching algorithms. This will presumably further strengthen the relative importance and value of HLA matching in keratoplasty, it will enforce the demand for matched corneas and it will call for continuous adaptation of our allocation criteria.

Trends in the Demand for Corneal Allografts at BIS

The latest change in the demand is characterized by the fact that the number of patients on the BIS waiting list who are typed for HLA class I *plus* II, i.e. for whom the new and more promising way is sought, has increased to 76%, while recipients for whom only a class I match is required, i.e. for whom only the old way is sought, decreased to 24%. This will force us to care for complete class I and II typing of almost every corneal donor very soon.

On the other hand, there are also categories of patients who can less well be served with an optimal HLA match. These are e.g. homozygous patients, patients with multiple specific antibodies after previous immune rejections and patients with rather rare tissue typing. If a reliable calculation of their presumed waiting time is still possible and delivers an acceptable waiting time, then these patients can, of course, be incorporated into a graded allocation system which pays proper attention to the special needs of such patients with restricted matching chances [9, 11]. If a matching chance in such a case, however, seems practically to be zero then such patients must accept random transplants and seek protection against immune reactions from all available medical immunosuppressive support.

Thus, BIS will continuously be confronted with the need to adjust and specify its international allocation criteria not only to the scientific progress in this field but also to the special needs of special patients in order to serve them best.

Conclusion

The new results and prospects of improved HLA matching are important for all ophthalmologists and their keratoplasty patients, but also for BIS as an international service center for the allocation of corneal grafts. BIS will continuously adjust its allocation criteria in such a way that new scientific results and items are properly reflected. One such important item is the increasing demand from ophthalmologists to obtain a reliable prediction on the waiting time for a defined matching grade as elaborated on in this volume by Böhringer et al. [9].

In order to improve the availability of HLA-typed as well as untyped corneas for transplantation, it is also necessary to further increase donor recruitment activities, especially in Germany. It has been BIS' policy to help in such activities as intensively as possible with its experience.

There is no principal reason for a lasting general shortage in donor corneas in our countries, and neither is there a reason for a principal shortage in typed donor corneas. If science has found out that typed and well-matched corneas are advantageous for most patients, then we will find ways to supply these corneas within short time adequately.

References

1   Sundmacher R, Reinhard T: Überwindung des Engpasses. Dtsch Ärztebl 2000;20:1452–1455.
2   BIS Foundation (Bio Implant Services Foundation), Annual Reports, Leiden, The Netherlands, 1998–1999.
3   Claas FHJ, Roelen DL, D'Amaro J, Völker-Dieben HJ: The role of HLA in corneal transplantation; in Zierhut M (ed): Immunology of Corneal Transplantation. Buren/NL, Aeolus Press, 1994, p 47.
4   Völker-Dieben HJ, D'Amaro J, de Lange P: Interaction between prognostic factors for corneal allograft survival. Transplant Proc 1989;21:3135.

5 Vail A, Gore SM, Bradley BA, Easty DL, Rogers CA, Armitage WJ: Conclusions of the corneal transplantation follow-up study. Br J Ophthalmol 1997;81:631.

6 Sanfilippo F, MacQuenn JM, Vaughn WK, Foulks GN: Reduced graft rejection with good HLA-A and -B matching in high-risk corneal transplantation. N Engl J Med 1986;315:29.

7 Schipper RF: Population genetic parameters of the HLA system: Methods and applications; Dissertation, Leiden 1996.

8 Völker-Dieben HJ, D'Amaro J, Kok van Alphen CC: Hierarchy of prognostic factors for corneal allograft survival. Aust NZ J Ophthalmol 1987;15:11.

9 Böhringer D, Reinhard T, Böhringer S, Enczmann J, Godehard E, Sundmacher R: Predicting waiting time on the waiting list for HLA-matched corneal grafts. Tissue Antigens 2002;59: 407–411.

10 Reinhard T, Böhringer D, Enczmann J, Kögler G, Mayweg S, Wernet P, Sundmacher R: Improvement of graft prognosis in penetrating normal-risk keratoplasty by HLA class I and II matching; in Sundmacher R (ed): Adequate HLA Matching in Keratoplasty. Dev Ophthalmol. Basel, Karger, 2003, vol 36, pp 42–49.

11 Persijn GG, Smits J, De Meester J, Frei U: Three year experience with the new Eurotransplant Kidney Allocation System 1996–1999, Transplantation Proceedings, 33, 821–823, 2001.

12 Völker-Dieben HJ, Claas F, D'Amaro J, et al: Beneficial effect of HLA-DR matches on the survival of corneal allografts. Transplantation 2000;70:640–648.

13 Richtlinien zum Führen einer Hornhautbank. Dtsch Ärztebl 2000(Aug);31–32.

T.M.M.H. de By, MBA
BIS Foundation, POB 2304
NL–2301 CH Leiden (The Netherlands)
Tel. +31 715 795712 , Fax +31 715 790903, E-Mail theodeby@bisfoundation.nl

Sundmacher R (ed): Adequate HLA Matching in Keratoplasty.
Dev Ophthalmol. Basel, Karger, 2003, vol 36, pp 62–73

....

Future HLA Matching Strategies in Clinical Transplantation

*Frans H.J. Claas, Dave L. Roelen, Machteld Oudshoorn,
Ilias I.N. Doxiadis*

Department of Immunohaematology and Blood Transfusion, Leiden University
Medical Center and Europdonor, Leiden, The Netherlands

Abstract

Background: HLA matching has shown to be beneficial in clinical transplantation. Due
to the enormous polymorphism of the HLA system, however, it is not feasible to select a
completely HLA-matched donor for every potential recipient. Only for patients with frequently
occurring HLA phenotypes is it realistic to expect a well-matched donor within a reasonable
waiting time. The majority of patients will be transplanted with a partially mismatched donor. In
order to select the optimal donor for this category of patients, it is important to take advantage of
the differential immunogenicity and thus differential importance of mismatched HLA antigens.

Methods: Based on retrospective analyses of graft survival data and in vitro tests
measuring T-cell alloreactivity, the relative importance of different mismatches was evaluated.

Results: It has been possible to define acceptable or permissible mismatches
with a low immunogenicity, which are associated with a good graft survival, versus taboo
mismatches with a high immunogenicity and a poor graft survival.

Conclusions: Further developing this new line of permissible versus taboo
mismatches, a new strategy will emerge for future HLA matching, which will not only suit
a rare number of patients with frequent haplotypes but a great percentage of all patients. This
principle of different immunogenicity of different mismatches can not only be applied to
T-cell alloreactivity as shown here, but also to B-cell alloreactivity, where a recently developed computer algorithm (HLA matchmaker) can be instrumental in selecting donors with
HLA mismatches, which do not lead to alloantibody formation.

Introduction

It is generally accepted that HLA matching of donor and recipient has
a beneficial effect in clinical transplantation [1]. This is due to the fact that

confrontation with allogeneic cells and tissue lead to both humoral and cellular immune responses which are directly responsible for complications such as graft rejection and, in case of bone marrow or stem cell transplantation, graft-versus-host disease [1, 2].

HLA matching is not only considered important in organ and stem cell transplantation, but also in corneal keratoplasty. Despite the fact that the eye is often considered to be an immunologically privileged site, a beneficial effect of HLA matching has been described both for high- and low-risk corneal transplants [3, 4]. The far majority of these detrimental alloimmune responses are directed against foreign HLA molecules, but also minor histocompatibility antigens may serve as targets. The best way to prevent alloimmune reactions leading to rejection is to select donors which share all histocompatibility antigens with the recipient.

The only optimal donor recipient combination is a monozygotic twin pair. In all other situations, individuals are mismatched for histocompatibility antigens and alloimmune responses are likely to occur. Considering the dominance of the major histocompatibility antigens, selection of HLA identical siblings or HLA identical unrelated donors may prevent a severe alloimmune response, although complete HLA matching is not a guarantee that no destructive immune reactions will take place.

In the family situation, the chance to find a completely HLA identical donor is about 30%. However, to find an HLA identical unrelated donor is very difficult due to the enormous polymorphism of the HLA system. The recent introduction of molecular typing techniques has even increased the complexity of the HLA system. Some of the serologically defined HLA antigens can now be subdivided in many different alleles, for instance of the serologically defined HLA-A2 antigen where more than 50 different alleles have been described [5].

The practical implications of the complexity of the HLA system for the selection of HLA-matched unrelated donors are well illustrated by the international efforts to establish a large pool of potential stem cell donors. Even with more than 7 million HLA-typed potential donors available, it is for many leukemia patients and especially for non-Caucasoid patients with rare HLA types, impossible to find a matched donor [6]. Therefore it is not realistic to aim at finding a completely HLA-matched unrelated donor for most of the potential transplant recipients taking into a consideration that the donor pool for potential kidney or corneal transplant recipients is far smaller than the one for potential stem cell recipients.

Our strategy for donor selection has to change from structural matching (donor and recipient must have exactly the same HLA molecules) to functional matching (the immune system of the recipient should not react strongly to the selected (mismatched) donor or, in case of bone marrow transplantation, the donor should not make a vigorous immune response to the recipient). In principle there are two approaches to determine which donor recipient combinations will meet the criteria of a functionally matched combination. One of the ways to analyze the immunogenicity of the different HLA mismatches is by retrospective analyses of graft survival data. Another approach is to monitor the alloimmune response of the patient in vitro with functional assays that can predict the presence or absence of an in vivo immune response by alloreactive T or B lymphocytes [7]. The possibilities of these approaches are discussed in this review.

Acceptable and Taboo Mismatches in Clinical Transplantation

Retrospective analyses of graft survival data have shown that the immunogenicity of HLA mismatches may differ enormously. One of the conclusions of such studies is that the HLA phenotype of recipient, and especially the HLA-DR antigens, may be predictive for a weak or strong alloimmune response. Transplantation of HLA mismatched kidney grafts in high responders will lead to a very poor graft survival while transplantation of mismatched grafts in low responders will result in a good graft survival.

On the basis of such analyses, HLA-DR6-positive recipients have been described to be high responders [5] whereas HLA-DR1-positive recipients have suggested to be low responders [8]. Similar studies, but now looking at the specific HLA mismatches of the donor, have shown that some HLA-DR mismatches are more immunogenic than others. For instance, kidney grafts from donors mismatched for HLA-DR6 are less immunogenic than grafts from donors with other HLA-DR mismatches [9]. However, both the data on the association of a particular HLA-DR antigen of the recipient with the strength of an alloimmune response and the data on the differential immunogenicity of particular HLA mismatches of the donor have not been confirmed in all studies. More recent studies suggest that the immunogenicity of an HLA mismatch should be considered in the context of the patients' own HLA phenotype. On the basis of these types of studies, Maruya et al. [10] were able to define so-called permissible HLA mismatches. Grafts mismatched for permissible HLA class I antigens have a similar graft survival as completely HLA identical grafts. Similarly, Vereerstraeten et al. [11] were able to define permissible and detrimental HLA-DR mismatches. The usefulness of this approach was also demonstrated in a study by Doxiadis et al. [12], who could demonstrate that certain HLA class I mismatches were highly immunogenic in patients with some HLA phenotypes and not in patients with another phenotype. For instance, survival of kidney grafts with a single HLA-B7 mismatch was significantly

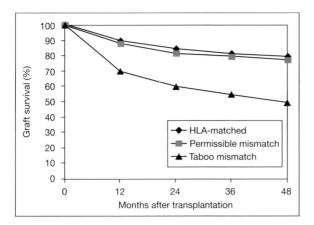

Fig. 1. Graft survival of completely HLA-matched kidney grafts and grafts mismatched for a single HLA antigen. Taboo mismatches have a very poor graft survival while permissible (or acceptable) mismatches have a similar graft survival as completely HLA-matched donors [based on references 10–12].

lower in patients which were HLA-A1-positive (45% after 5 years) compared to HLA-A1-negative recipients (75% after 5 years). These studies have led to the definition of so-called taboo mismatches: specific HLA mismatches which lead to a very poor graft survival and which should be avoided.

A problem is that permissible and taboo mismatches are defined by a better or poorer graft survival when groups of patients are compared (fig. 1), whereas a permissible or taboo mismatch has no direct implication for an individual patient. Both in the group of patients with taboo mismatches and in the group of patients with permissible mismatches, some patients reject early while other patients have an excellent graft survival.

Similar population studies showed that the immunogenicity of the non-inherited maternal HLA antigens (NIMA) is lower than that of the non-inherited paternal HLA antigens (NIPA) [13]. Both renal transplant studies and bone marrow transplantation data show that mismatches for NIMA lead to a significantly kidney graft survival [14] and a significantly lower incidence of graft-versus-host disease compared to grafts with NIPA mismatches [15]. But also here, NIMA or NIPA mismatches are not a guarantee for excellent survival or complications for an individual patient.

In conclusion, studies on the population level can only give an indication of the chance that graft survival in case of a particular HLA mismatch is good or bad. Other parameters are necessary to select the optimal (mismatched) donor for an individual patient.

In vitro Analysis of Alloreactive T Cells

As T cells are considered to play an essential and important role in graft rejection, it is attractive to select a donor on the basis of a low T-cell alloreactivity of the patient to the HLA mismatches of the donor.

For more than 25 years, the mixed lymphocyte culture (MLC) and the cell-mediated lympholysis (CML) test have been used to monitor alloreactivity to respectively HLA class II and HLA class I mismatches in vitro. Several studies have shown a correlation between hyporesponsiveness in MLC or CML and long-term graft survival [16, 17]. However, other studies show that measurement of the MLC and CML responder's status has only a limited or no prognostic value [18, 19]. The main problem with these assays is the fact that they are not quantitative assays. Quantification of alloreactive T cells became possible with the introduction of limiting dilution analysis (LDA). With this approach it is possible to quantify both helper T-cell and cytotoxic T-cell precursor frequencies [20, 21]. The results obtained with these assays show that different individuals can have different T-cell precursor frequencies for the same HLA mismatches. Furthermore, in one individual, different T-cell precursor frequencies are found against different HLA alloantigens [22].

Studies on the population level have shown that the cytotoxic T lymphocyte precursor (CTLp) frequencies for HLA-B mismatches are significantly higher than CTLp frequencies against HLA-A [23]. A possible clinical relevance of these limiting dilution assays is suggested by the fact that in transplantation, mismatches for HLA-B seem to be more immunogenic and lead more often to graft rejection than mismatches for HLA-A.

A correlation between an increase of CTLp frequency and rejection of a kidney graft has been described [24], but other studies showed that high CTLp frequencies were also found in patients with a good graft function [25]. Nevertheless, a recent study showed that tapering of immunosuppression in renal transplant recipients is successful in case of low CTLp frequencies, whereas in case of high donor-specific CTLp frequencies, rejection often occurred [26]. Several studies showed that the CTLp frequency is predictive for the occurrence of graft-versus-host disease in unrelated bone marrow transplantation [27, 28], while the helper T-cell precursor frequency was found to be predictive in case of HLA identical sibling bone marrow transplantation [21, 29].

In our center, CTLp assays have been an integrated part of the search selection procedure as well. More recently, DNA-based typing for HLA class I became available. This allowed us to determine the correlation of CTLp frequencies directed against incompatibilities at the HLA-A, -B, and -C locus in 211 donor-recipient pairs [30]. HLA class I incompatibilities were associated with high CTLp frequencies. High CTLp frequencies were also seen in 14% of the HLA-A, -B and -C allele-matched pairs. These CTLs are probably directed to minor histocompatibility antigens. A low CTLp frequency occurred in 7% of the pairs mismatched for HLA-A or -B. The successful outcome of transplants performed in the latter cases suggest that the CTLp test can be used as a tool to detect permissible mismatches when no fully matched donor is available.

The clinical relevance of the CTLp assay can be increased by distinguishing the contribution of primed versus naive CTLs to the cytotoxic activity. Primed CTLs have a higher avidity for donor antigen and are resistant to anti-CD8 antibodies whereas the reactivity of naive CTLs is blocked by this antibody treatment [31].

These subtypes of CTLs can also be distinguished on the basis of their reactivity in the presence of cyclosporin A. Primed CTLs are more resistant to cyclosporin A compared to naive CTLs [32]. Extensive studies in heart transplantation recipients, both looking at the peripheral blood and graft infiltrating cells, showed that rejection of a graft is not associated with an increased CTLp frequency but with an increased frequency of primed donor-specific CTLs [33]. Similar data were also found for the rejection of corneal transplants [34]. Furthermore, rejection of heart transplants was associated with the resistance of CD4-positive T cells direct against mismatched HLA class II antigens of the donor for antibodies against CD4 [35]. All these studies concerned monitoring of patients after transplantation.

Although some studies suggest a clinical relevance for LDA assays detecting T-helper cells (based on quantification of the number of IL-2-producing cells), most studies do not find a direct association between the helper T-cell frequency and the clinical course of an organ transplant. This is not surprising considering the different types of CD4-positive T cells which may become activated after recognition of a foreign HLA class II molecule. Some of these T cells recognize the alloantigens via direct recognition (donor antigens presented by donor antigen presenting cells) while others recognize peptides derived from donor alloantigens in the context of self MHC on autologous antigen presenting cells of the patient (indirect recognition). The presence of the latter type of CD4-positive T cells was found to be associated with the occurrence of chronic rejection [36, 37]. More recent studies are focussing on the relevance of the genetically determined cytokine polymorphisms [38, 39] and/or the levels of cytokines produced by donor-specific alloreactive T cells [40] and by this try to find other parameters associated with graft rejection or transplantation tolerance.

The old concept that Th1 responses are associated with graft rejection and Th2 responses are associated with a good graft survival was too simple and is not supported by the actual data. Graft rejecting can also occur on the basis of an alloimmune response by Th2 cells [41]. One of the ways by which the immune system can prevent a detrimental alloimmune response is by the activity of regulatory T cells which are able to downregulate the alloimmune response leading to rejection [42, 43]. Although several types of CD4-positive regulatory T cells are characterized, which are able to downregulate an alloimmune response in vitro and/or in vivo in rodents, the most striking data so far in the field of clinical transplantation are those published by Suciu-Foca and co-workers [44], who showed that an excellent graft survival is associated with the presence of CD8-positive, CD28-negative regulatory T cells. These cells seem to be able to modulate the antigen presenting capacity of dendritic cells in such a way that CD4-positive cells cannot be activated anymore [45]. Monitoring patients for the presence of these CD8-positive regulatory cells seems to be a suitable tool to select those people who have a very low chance to reject their graft. However, so far this is only possible after transplantation as these CD8-positive regulatory cells are induced by the transplant in the presence of immunosuppressive drugs.

Although some of the in vitro studies on the T-cell allorepertoire of a patient are promising, we do not have a suitable tool available yet to predict before the transplantation which patient will develop a detrimental cellular alloimmune response and which patient will hardly recognize the mismatched histocompatibility antigens on the graft. Furthermore, these assays are very labor-intensive and cannot be performed in a routine setting for all patients.

Tools to Predict the Alloimmune Response by B Lymphocytes

Next to alloreactive T cells, alloantibodies produced after activation of B lymphocytes, may play a crucial role in graft rejection. Since the introduction of more sensitive assays to measure donor-specific alloantibodies, it becomes more and more clear that graft rejection is often associated with antibody formation [46, 47]. Until recently it was not possible to predict against which HLA mismatch a patient will produce alloantibodies and against which HLA mismatch the chance of antibody formation is almost zero.

Several studies suggest that transplantation with HLA mismatches which belong to a cross-reactive group (CREG) with the patient's own HLA antigens give a lower chance for antibody induction [48, 49]. However, transplantation with a donor carrying cross-reactive antigens is not a guarantee that no antibodies will be formed and certainly not a guarantee that alloreactive T cells do not react [50].

An alternative approach would be the development of a functional test like the one described for the quantification of alloreactive T cells. Indeed,

Mulder et al. [51] were able to develop a B-cell precursor assay on the basis of which one can determine the frequency of B cells that are able to produce specific antibodies against a particular HLA mismatch. However, so far this assay was mainly successful in patients which were already immunized and had circulating antibodies in their serum. As only very low frequencies of alloreactive B lymphocytes were found in non-immunized individuals, this assay does not seem to have a predictive value for the situation after transplantation or transfusion.

A very promising tool however is the recently developed computer program called HLA matchmaker [52], which is a molecularly based algorithm to define acceptable mismatches for highly sensitized patients. The algorithm is based on the concept that immunogenic epitopes are represented by amino acid triplets on those parts of the HLA molecules that are accessible for alloantibodies. The principle of the program is that the patient does not make antibody to self triplets. By both intra- and interlocus comparisons of triplets present on the patient's own HLA antigens and a mismatched HLA antigen, it can predict the immunogenicity of that particular mismatch [53]. If no triplet mismatches are present, the patient is supposed not to make alloantibodies.

Recently, we have validated this theoretical concept by checking the prediction of this program with the extensive screening and cross-match tests routinely performed to define acceptable mismatches for highly sensitized patients. These studies showed that in case of HLA mismatched donors with 0 triplet mismatches, no alloantibodies are found. Even more interesting was the fact that HLA alloantigens with only 1 triplet mismatch are also hardly immunogenic. These data suggest that the HLA matchmaker concept can indeed be used to predict the absence of antibody induction in case of particular HLA mismatches.

Epilogue

Since the introduction of molecular HLA typing techniques the number of HLA alleles has increased almost exponentially. Considering the polymorphism of the HLA system, it is not realistic to aim at and wait for an HLA identical donor for every potential transplant recipient. Only for patients with a frequently occurring HLA phenotype can one hope to receive a fully HLA-matched organ or corneal allograft within a reasonable waiting time. However, we should consider an alternative strategy for most of the patients to select the most suitable donor.

Considering the important role of alloreactive T and B cells in graft rejection, our strategy should focus on the selection of donors with HLA mismatches that are hardly immunogenic for the immune system of the specific patient.

On the population level the immunogenicity of particular HLA mismatches can be determined on the basis of retrospective analyses of graft survival data. Such studies have indeed led to the identification of so-called acceptable or permissible mismatches. Graft survival in case of a donor organ with such a mismatch is almost similar to graft survival of a completely HLA identical donor.

Another approach is the inventory of the alloimmune repertoire of an individual patient. In vitro studies show that the immune response to a foreign HLA antigen may differ enormously. Especially the analysis of the cytotoxic T-cell repertoire has been useful in this respect. In contrast, no suitable in vitro assays are available to predict the alloimmune response by B lymphocytes. However, on the basis of the HLA matchmaker concept, it seems possible to predict which HLA mismatches do not lead to alloantibody formation. It would be convenient if a similar type of approach could be used for the prediction of an alloimmune response by T lymphocytes. The problem is that T-cell recognition is far more complicated than the situation for alloantibody formation. The current matchmaker program only considers polymorphic epitopes on antibody accessible sites of the HLA molecules and does not consider the polymorphism within the groove which is mainly recognized by alloreactive T cells.

Considering the fact that alloreactive T cells indirectly recognize these polymorphisms on the basis of peptides present in the groove of the HLA molecules makes it unlikely that adaptation of the HLA matchmaker program for T-cell recognition is a simple procedure. For the time being it is essential to develop additional and more specific in vitro assays to predict the alloreactive T-cell response in vivo.

In conclusion, selection of a completely HLA identical donor should only be considered for patients with frequently occurring HLA phenotypes. In all other situations we should use strategies aiming at functional matching defined as a low immunogenicity of the donor mismatches for the immune system of the recipient.

Acknowledgements

This work was supported by grants of the J.A. Cohen Institute for Radiation Protection (IRS) and the Dutch Kidney Foundation. Ingrid Claproth is acknowledged for excellent secretarial help.

References

1   Opelz G, Wujciak T, Dohler B, Scherer S, Mytilineos J: HLA compatibility and organ transplant survival. Collaborative Transplant Study. Rev Immunogenet 1999;1:334–342.

2   Mickelson EM, Petersdorf E, Anasetti C, Martin P, Woolfrey A, Hansen JA: HLA matching in hematopoietic cell transplantation. Hum Immunol 2000;61:92–100.

3   Völker-Dieben HJ, Claas FHJ, Schreuder GMT, Schipper RF, Pels E, Persijn GG, Smits J, D'Amaro J: Beneficial effect of HLA-DR matching the survival of corneal allografts. Transplantation 2000; 70:640–648.

4   Boisjoly HM, Roy R, Bernard PM, Dube I, Laughrea PA, Bazin R: Association between corneal graft reactions and HLA compatibility. Ophthalmology 1990;97:1689–1696.

5   Robinson J, Waller MJ, Parham P, Bodmer JG, Marsh SG: IMGT/HLA database – A sequence database for the human major histocompatibility complex. Tissue Antigens 2000;55:280–287.

6   Oudshoorn M, Cornelissen JJ, Fibbe WE, De Graef-Meeder ER, Lie JL, Schreuder GMT, Sintnicolaas K, Willemze R, Vossen JM, Van Rood JJ: Problems and possible solutions in finding an unrelated bone marrow donor. Results of consecutive searches for 240 Dutch patients. Bone Marrow Transplant 1997;20:1011–1017.

7   Hendriks GFJ, Schreuder GMT, Claas FHJ, D'Amaro J, Persijn GG, Cohen B, Van Rood JJ: HLA-DRw6 and renal allograft rejection. Br Med J 1983;286:85–87.

8   Cook DJ, Cecka JM, Terasaki PI: HLA-DR1 recipients have the highest kidney graft survival. Transplant Proc 1987;18:675–677.

9   Hendriks GFJ, D'Amaro J, Persijn GG, Schreuder GMT, Lansbergen Q, Cohen B, Van Rood JJ: Excellent outcome after transplantation of renal allografts from HLA-DRw6-positive donors even in HLA-DR mismatches. Lancet 1983;ii:187–189.

10 Maruya E, Takemoto S, Terasaki PI: HLA matching: Identification of permissible HLA mismatches. Clin Transplant 1993;5:11–20.

11 Vereerstraeten P, Dupont E, Andrien M, De Pauw L, Abranowicz D, Goldman M, Kinnaert P: Influence of donor-recipient HLA-DR mismatches and OKT3 prophylaxis on cadaver kidney transplantation. Transplantation 1995;60:253–258.

12 Doxiadis IIN, Smits JMA, Schreuder GMT, Persijn GG, Van Houwelingen HC, Van Rood JJ, Claas FHJ, et al: Association between specific HLA combinations and probability of kidney allograft loss: The taboo concept. Lancet 1996;348:850–853.

13 Van Rood JJ, Claas FHJ: Both self and non-inherited maternal HLA antigens influence the immune response. Immunol Today 2000;21:269–273.

14 Burlingham WJ, Grailer AD, Heisey DM, Claas FHJ, Norman D, Mohannkumar T, Brennan DC, De Fijter H, Van Gelder T, Pirsch JD, Sollinger HW, Bean MA: The effect of tolerance to non-inherited maternal HLA antigens on the survival of renal transplants from sibling donors. N Engl J Med 1998;339:1657–1664.

15 Van Rood JJ, Loberiza FR, Zhang MH, Oudshoorn M, Claas F, Cairo MS, Champlin RE, Gale RP, Ringden O, Hows JM, Horowitz MH: The effect of tolerance to non-inherited maternal antigens (NIMA) on the occurrence of graft-versus-host disease after bone marrow transplantation from a parent or HLA identical sibling. Blood 2002;99:1572–1577.

16 Goulmy E, Persijn G, Paul LC, Wilmink J, Van Rood JJ: HLA regulates postrenal transplant CML non-reactivity. J Immunol 1985;135:3082–3086.

17 Reinsmoen NL, Kaufman D, Matas AJ, Sutherland D, Najarian JJ, Bach FH: A new in vitro approach to determine acquired tolerance in long-term kidney allograft recipients. Transplantation 1990;50:783–790.

18 Goulmy E, Stijnen T, Groenewoud AF, Persijn GG, Blokland E, Pool J, Paul LC, Van Rood JJ: Renal transplant patients monitored by the cell-mediated lympholysis assay. Evaluation of its clinical value. Transplantation 1989;48:559–563.

19 Pfeffer PF, Thorsby E, Hirschberg H: Donor-specific decreased cell-mediated cytotoxicity in recipients of well-functioning, one HLA haplotype mismatched kidney allografts. Transplantation 1983;35:546–551.

20 Lindahl KF, Wilson DD: Histocompatibility antigen activated cytotoxic T lymphocytes. II. Estimates of the frequency and specificity of precursors. J Exp Med 1977;145:508–522.

21 Theobald M, Nierle T, Bunjes D, Arnold R, Heimpel H: Host-specific interleukin-2 secreting donor T-cell precursors as predictors of acute graft-versus-host disease in bone marrow transplantation between HLA identical siblings. N Engl J Med 1992;327:1613–1617.

22   Zhang L, Li SG, Vandekerkckhove B, Termijtelen A, Van Rood JJ, Claas FHJ: Analysis of cytotoxic T cell precursor frequencies directed against individual HLA-A- and -B alloantigens. J Immunol Methods 1989;121:39–45.

23   Zhang L, Van Bree S, Van Rood JJ, Claas FHJ: The effect of individual HLA-A and -B mismatches on the generation of cytotoxic T lymphocyte precursors. Transplantation 1990;50:1008–1010.

24   Herzog WR, Zanker B, Irschick EU, Huber C, Franz HE, Wagner H, Kabelitz D: Selective reduction of donor-specific cytotoxic T lymphocyte precursors in patients with a well-functioning kidney allograft. Transplantation 1987;43:384–389.

25   Steinmann J, Leimenstoll G, Engemann R, Weyand M, Westphal E, Müller-Ruchholtz W: Clinical relevance of cytotoxic T cell precursor (p-CTL) frequencies in allograft recipients. Transplant Proc 1990;22:1873.

26   Van Besouw NM, Van der Mast BJ, De Kuiper P, Smak-Gregoor PJ, Vaessen LM, Ijzermans JN, Van Gelder T, Weimar W: Donor-specific T-cell reactivity identifies kidney transplant patients in whom immunosuppressive therapy can be safely reduced. Transplantation 2000;70:136–143.

27   Kaminski E, Hows J, Man S, Brookes P, Mackinnan S, Hughes T, Avakian O, Goldman JM, Batchelor JR: Prediction of graft-versus-host disease by frequency analysis of cytotoxic T cells after unrelated donor bone marrow transplantation. Transplantation 1989;48:608–613.

28   Roosnek E, Hogendijk S, Zawadynski S, Speiser D, Tiercy JM, Helg C, Chapuis B, Gratwohl A, Gmur J, Seger R: The frequency of pretransplant donor cytotoxic T cell precursors with anti-host specificity predicts survival of patients transplanted with bone marrow from donors other than HLA-identical siblings. Transplantation 1993;56:691–696.

29   Weston LE, Geczy AF, Farrell C: Donor helper T cell frequencies as predictors of acute graft-versus-host disease in bone marrow transplantation between HLA identical siblings. Transplantation 1997;64:836–841.

30   Oudshoorn M, Doxiadis IIN, Van den Berg-Loonen PM, Voorter CEM, Verduyn W, Claas FHJ: Functional versus structural matching: Can the CTLp test be replaced by HLA allele typing? Hum Immunol 2002;63:176–184.

31   Roelen D, Datema G, Van Bree S, Zhang L, Van Rood J, Claas F: Evidence that antibody formation against a certain HLA alloantigen is associated not with a quantitative but with a qualitative change in the cytotoxic T cells recognizing the same antigen. Transplantation 1992; 53:899–903.

32   Roelen DL, Van Bree FP, Schanz U, Van Rood JJ, Claas FH: Differential inhibition of primed alloreactive CTLs in vitro by clinically used concentrations of cylosporine and FK506. Transplantation 1993;56:190–195.

33   Ouwehand AJ, Baan CC, Roelen DL, Vaessen LM, Balk AH, Jutte NM, Bos E, Claas FHJ, Weimar W: The detection of cytotoxic T cells with high-affinity receptors for donor antigens in the transplanted heart as a prognostic factor for graft rejection. Transplantation 1993;56:1223–1229.

34   Roelen DL, Van Beelen E, Van Bree SP, Van Rood JJ, Völker-Dieben HJ, Claas FH: The presence of activated donor HLA class I reactive T lymphocytes is associated with rejection of corneal grafts. Transplantation 1995;59:1039–1042.

35   Van Emmerik NE, Loonen EH, Vaessen LM, Balk AH, Mochtar B, Claas FHJ, Weimar W: The avidity, not the mere presence, of primed cytotoxic T lymphocytes for donor human leukocyte class II antigens determines their clinical relevance after heart transplantation. J Heart Lung Transplant 1997;16:240–249.

36   Ciubotariu R, Liu Z, Colovai AI, Ho E, Iteseu S, Ravalli S, Hardy MA, Cortesini R, Rose EA, Suciu Foca N: Persistent allopeptide reactivity and epitope spreading in chronic rejection of organ allografts. J Clin Invest 1998;101:398–405.

37   SivaSai KS, Smith MA, Poindexter NH, Sundaresan SR, Trudock EP, Lynch SP, Cooper SD, Patterson GA, Mohanakumar T: Indirect recognition of donor HLA class I peptides in lung transplant recipients with bronchiolitis obliterans syndrome. Transplantation 1999;67:1094–1098.

38   Turner D, Grant SC, Yonan N, Sheldon S, Dyer PA, Sinnott PJ, Hutchinson IV: Cytokine gene polymorphism and heart transplant rejection. Transplantation 1997;64:776–779.

39   Asderakis A, Sankaran D, Dyer P, Johnson RW, Pravica V, Sinnot PJ, Roberts I, Hutchinson IV: Association of polymorphisms in the human interferon-γ and interleukin-10 gene with acute and

chronic kidney transplant outcome: The cytokine effect on transplantation. Transplantation 2001; 71:674–677.

40 Najafian N, Salama AD, Fedoseyeva EV, Benichou G, Sayegh MH: Enzyme-linked immunosorbent spot assay analysis of peripheral blood lymphocyte reactivity to donor HLA-DR peptides: Potential novel assay for prediction of outcomes for renal transplant recipients. J Am Soc Nephrol 2002;13:252–259.

41 Zelenika D, Adams E, Humm S, Lin CY, Waldmann H, Cobbold SP: The role of CD4+ T-cell subsets in determining transplantation rejection or tolerance. Immunol Rev 2001;182:164–179.

42 Kingsley CI, Karim M, Bushell AR, Wood KJ: CD25+CD4+ regulatory T cells prevent graft rejection: CTLA-4- and IL-10-dependent immunoregulation of alloresponses. J Immunol 2002;168: 1080–1086.

43 Gregori S, Casorati M, Amuchastegui S, Smiroldo S, Davalli AM, Adorini L: Regulatory T cells induced by 1α,25-dihydroxyvitamin D₃ and mycophenolate mofetil treatment mediate transplantation tolerance. J Immunol 2001;167:1945–1953.

44 Chang CC, Ciubotariu R, Manavalan JS, Yuan J, Colovai AI, Piazza F, Lederman S, Colonna M, Cortesini R, Dalla-Favera R, Suciu-Foca N: Tolerization of dendritic cells by TS cells: The crucial role of inhibitory receptors ILT3 and ILT4. Nat Immunol 2002;3:237–243.

45 Liu Z, Tugulea S, Cortesini R, Suciu-Foca N: Specific suppression of T-helper alloreactivity by allo-MHC class I restricted CD8+CD28− T cells. Int Immunol 1998;10:775–783.

46 McKenna RM, Takemoto SK, Terasaki PI: Anti-HLA antibodies after solid organ transplantation. Transplantation 2000;69:319–326.

47 Christiaans MH, Nieman F, Van Hooff JP, Van den Berg-Loonen EM: Detection of HLA class I and II antibodies by ELISA and complement-dependent cytotoxicity before and after transplantation. Transplantation 2000;69:917–927.

48 Rodey GE, Neylan JF, Whelchel JD, Revels KW, Bray RA: Epitope specificity of HLA class I alloantibodies. I. Frequency analysis of antibodies to private versus public specificities in potential transplant recipients. Hum Immunol 1994;39:272–280.

49 Papassavas AC, Iniotaki-Theodoraki A, Boletis J, Kostakis A, Stavropoulous-Giokas C: Epitope analysis of HLA class I donor specific antibodies in sensitized renal transplant recipients. Transplantation 2000;70:323–327.

50 Stobbe I, Van der Meer-Prins EMW, De Lange P, Oudshoorn M, Doxiadis IIN, Claas FHJ: In vitro CTL precursor frequencies do not reflect a beneficial effect of cross-reactive group (CREG) matching. Hum Immunol 2000;61:879–883.

51 Mulder A, Kardol MJ, Kamp J, Uit Het Broek C, Schreuder GMT, Doxiadis IIN, Claas FHJ: Determination of the frequency of HLA antibody secreting B lymphocytes in alloantigen-sensitized individuals. Clin Exp Immunol 2001;124:9–15.

52 Duquesnoy RJ: HLA matchmaker: A molecularly based donor selection algorithm for highly alloimmunized patients. Transplant Proc 2001;33:493–497.

53 Duquesnoy RJ: HLA matchmaker. I. A molecularly based donor selection algorithm for highly alloimmunized patients. Hum Immunol 2002;63:299–352.

Frans H.J. Claas, Leiden University Medical Center,
Department of Immunohaematology and Blood Transfusion,
POB 9600, NL–2300 RC Leiden (The Netherlands)
Tel. +31 71 5263800, Fax +31 71 5216751, E-Mail fhjclaas@lumc.nl

Sundmacher R (ed): Adequate HLA Matching in Keratoplasty.
Dev Ophthalmol. Basel, Karger, 2003, vol 36, pp 74–88

....

The Role of Minor Histocompatibility Alloantigens in Penetrating Keratoplasty

J. Wayne Streilein, Carolina Arancibia-Caracamo, Hideya Osawa

Schepens Eye Research Institute, Department of Ophthalmology,
Harvard Medical School, Boston, Mass., USA

Abstract

Background/Aims: To review the experimental evidence that implicates minor histo-compatibility (H) antigens in the vulnerability of orthotopic corneal transplants to rejection, and to speculate on the possible role of minor H antigens in penetrating keratoplasty in humans.

Methods: Orthotopic corneal transplantations have been conducted in numerous inbred strains of mice and rats, and the fate of these grafts, as well as the immune responses mounted by recipients, have been examined in vivo and in vitro.

Results: Minor H antigens have been found to be more important barriers to the success of orthotopic corneal transplants in rodents than have grafts disparate at the major histocompatibility complex (MHC). The reasons for this reversal of the immunogenetic rules of transplantation reflect unique features of the cornea with respect to (a) expression of MHC-encoded molecules, (b) content of class II MHC-bearing antigen presenting cells, (c) vulnerability to rejection by direct alloreactive T cells, and (d) existence of ocular immune privilege.

Conclusion: Since minor H antigens are the major barriers to acceptance of orthotopic corneal allografts in rodents, minor H antigens should be considered as important targets of rejection in failed penetrating keratoplasty in humans.

Copyright © 2003 S. Karger AG, Basel

Discovery of Transplantation Antigens

Sixty years ago, Medawar [1] demonstrated that immune responses directed at so-called transplantation antigens on solid tissue allografts are responsible for graft rejection. Within the succeeding decade it became clear from studies on genetically inbred strains of rats and mice that (a) transplantation antigens are encoded by polymorphic alleles, (b) numerous gene loci encode different transplantation antigens, and (c) some transplantation antigens are stronger than others [2]. The last realization gave rise to the notion that there are major and minor histocompatibility (H) antigens. During the 1960s, numerous investigators contributed to the concept that a major histocompatibility complex (MHC) exists in each mammalian species, and that this unique chromosomal region encodes very strong transplantation antigens, termed class I and class II. Unlike minor H antigens, class I and II MHC antigens can be detected by antibody reagents and in vitro assays, making it possible to tissue type individuals. By the early 1970s it was possible to demonstrate that human recipients of solid organ allografts that were matched for class I and class II MHC antigens with the graft donor were much more likely to accept their grafts than recipients that were MHC mismatched with their donors. The fact that recipients of MHC-matched grafts still required systemic immunosuppression to secure graft survival indicates that minor H antigens (which cannot be matched at present by typing) are also important barriers to acceptance of solid tissue grafts. Since significantly less immunosuppression was needed to secure survival of MHC-matched grafts than MHC-mismatched grafts, there was general agreement that tissue typing for MHC gene products is beneficial to transplantation success [3].

Tissue Typing and Penetrating Keratoplasty Outcome

In humans, the MHC is termed HLA, and this chromosomal region encodes several class I (HLA-A, B, C) and class II (HLA-DP, DQ, DR) alloantigens. Cornea as a tissue expresses class I alloantigens, with epithelium expressing levels of class I antigen comparable to other tissues, and corneal endothelium expressing extremely low levels of class I alloantigens (see table 1) [4–7]. It was reported in 1979 [8] that MHC class II alloantigens are not expressed on any corneal cells under normal circumstances, with the exception of Langerhans cells at the limbus. Reduced MHC class I and absent MHC class II expression of cornea compared to other somatic tissues and organ anticipated difficulties in demonstrating that tissue typing might improve the fate of corneal transplants in humans. For the past 25 years the literature has been littered with studies claiming variably that HLA tissue matching either (a) promotes corneal transplant survival [9], or (b) fails to influence the fate of orthotopic corneal transplants [10–12]. Since penetrating keratoplasties suffer dramatically different outcomes depending upon whether the recipient eye is considered to be 'low-' or 'high-' risk, the literature of the past decade has been littered as well with studies claiming that HLA tissue matching (a) promotes

Table 1. Expression of MHC molecules on cornea and other solid tissue grafts

		Class I	Class II
Cornea (normal)	Epithelium	++	–
	Keratocytes	++	–
	Endothelium	+	–
	Dendritic cells and macrophages	++	–
Cornea (inflamed) or limbus	Epithelium	++++	–
	Keratocytes	+++	–
	Endothelium	++	–
	Dendritic cells and macrophages	++++	++++
Skin	Epidermis	+++	–
	Dermal fibroblasts	++	–
	Dendritic cells and macrophages	++++	++++
Kidney	Tubular epithelium	+++	–
	Stromal fibroblasts	++	–
	Dendritic cells and macrophages	+++	+++

+ = Intensity of expression, – = no expression – as judged by immunohistochemistry.

corneal transplant survival in high-risk eyes [13], or (b) fails to influence the fate of orthotopic corneal transplants in high-risk eyes [14–16]. In the somewhat acrimonious debate initiated by these disparate reports (the debate is illuminated in other chapters in this book), it is instructive to examine the results of recent basic research into the immunologic basis of orthotopic corneal transplantation rejection. From this examination, reasons emerge that offer at least partial explanation for the conundrum of tissue typing and corneal transplant outcome, and emphasize the unexpected importance of minor H antigens in dictating graft outcome.

Immunogenetics of Penetrating Keratoplasty in Laboratory Rodents

Since the late 1970s, experimentalists have developed the extraordinary technical skills required to carry out orthotopic corneal transplantation in inbred strains of rats and mice [17, 18]. This situation has dramatically changed our ability to analyze immune and immunogenetic factors governing the fate of corneal transplants. The clearest results bearing on the role of major and minor H antigens on cornea graft survival have emerged from studies in mice.

Originally reported by Sonoda and Streilein [18], and then confirmed by other laboratories [19], cornea grafts that confront their recipients with minor H antigens are much more likely to be rejected than grafts that confront their recipients with antigens encoded solely within the murine MHC, H-2 [18, 20]. For example, mice of the BALB/c strain reject 50% of corneas from minor H-incompatible B10.D2 donors, but less than 20% of corneas from MHC-only disparate BALB.B donors. Mice of the C57BL/6 strain reject 85% of corneas from minor H-only disparate BALB.B donors, but less than 50% of MHC-only disparate B10.D2 corneas [21]. The propensity for minor H-only disparate grafts to experience a higher rate of rejection than MHC-only disparate grafts also applies to corneas placed in high-risk eyes in mice [22].

Quite recently, Haskova et al. [23] have made the startling observation that cornea grafts from donors that differ from their recipients by only a *single* minor H disparity (H-3) are rejected at a high rate (approximately 70%) in low-risk eyes. This rejection incidence actually exceeds that of H-3-only incompatible skin grafts placed orthotopically. While the explanation of this observation is still to be deduced from ongoing experiments, this result strongly emphasizes the power of minor H antigens to promote cornea graft rejection.

The conclusion from these murine experiments is unavoidable: minor H antigens are much more significant barriers to cornea graft acceptance than antigens encoded by the MHC [24, 25]. Taken at face value, these results offer a simple explanation for the difficulty investigators and clinicians have encountered in trying to demonstrate that HLA typing and tissue matching can improve the fate of penetrating keratoplasties in humans. Contemporary tissue typing is incapable of matching donor and recipient for minor H antigens. If, as in experimental animals, these antigens are more important than MHC-encoded antigens in dictating the fate of human cornea grafts, then it is small wonder that HLA matching has such a small effect (if any) on cornea transplant success in the clinic.

One must admit, however, that the explanation offered above for the relative lack of influence of HLA matching on penetrating keratoplasty success in humans is only partially satisfying. If that explanation could lead to a greater understanding of the pathogenesis of cornea graft rejection, then the information might be turned to clinical advantage. Consequently, experimentalists have attempted to explain why minor H antigens are so important to cornea graft rejection in laboratory animals.

It is worth interjecting into the discussion at this point that the same evidence that implicates minor H antigens in promotion of cornea graft failure also points to an important role for immune privilege in cornea graft outcome.

BALB/c mice, that reject 50% of orthotopic C57BL/6 cornea grafts, accept the remaining 50% indefinitely! Similarly, C57BL/6 mice, that reject 85% of BALB.B cornea grafts, accept the remaining 15% indefinitely. No similar pattern exists in laboratory animals for orthotopic grafts of skin, heart or kidney. Grafts of other solid tissues that cross immunogenetic disparities of this magnitude are uniformly rejected – with no long-term survivors. It may well be that physiologic mechanisms that enable some cornea transplants to enjoy immune privilege in the eye are pertinent to the conclusion that minor H antigens are more important than MHC-encoded antigens in provoking cornea transplant rejection (see below).

Immune Effectors Elicited by Orthotopic Cornea Transplants in Laboratory Rodents

Upon recognition of foreign transplantation antigens on solid tissue and organ grafts, the immune system mounts a response that includes a diversity of effector cells and molecules [2]. Transplanters have demonstrated that allografts of skin, kidney, and heart (as examples) induce the formation of graft antigen-specific $CD4^+$ T cells (of the delayed hypersensitivity type), $CD8^+$ T cells (of the cytotoxic type), and humoral antibodies (of both complement fixing and non-fixing types). Whereas donor-specific antibodies formed in this manner usually fail to participate in acute and subacute graft rejection, these antibodies may contribute to the chronic rejection of solid tissue allografts. While antibodies are irrelevant to acute graft rejection, $CD4^+$ T cells alone have been shown to be capable of mediating acute rejection of solid organ transplants. Similarly, $CD8^+$ T cells alone can cause acute and subacute rejection of solid organ transplants. Thus, T cells are the exclusive mediators of acute allograft rejection.

When donor and recipient contain different alleles at the MHC and at multiple minor H loci, two distinct populations of responding T cells have been found to be activated [26] (see table 2). One population of T cells recognizes donor MHC-encoded antigens directly – cells of this type are called 'direct alloreactive T cells'. Another population of T cells recognizes peptides, derived from MHC and minor H alloantigenic proteins, that are loaded onto recipient-type MHC class I and class II molecules. These latter molecules are expressed on antigen presenting cells (APCs) of the recipient. Because this population of T cells only recognizes donor antigens via peptides expressed on self-MHC molecules, the responding T cells are called 'indirect alloreactive'. With respect to most solid tissue/organ transplants, rejection has been shown to be mediated by both 'direct' and 'indirect' alloreactive T cells.

Table 2. Diverse immune effectors in acute rejection of MHC plus minor H disparate solid tissue allografts

		Effectors responsible for acute rejection		
Graft	Site	CD4$^+$ T cells	CD8$^+$ T cells	Alloantibodies
Cornea	Low-risk eye	Yes (indirect[a] only)	No	No
Cornea	High-risk eye	Yes (direct[a] and indirect)	No	No
Skin	Orthotopic	Yes (direct and indirect)	Yes (direct and indirect)	No

[a]Direct and indirect refer to the type of allorecognition used by the effector T cells (see text).

A considerably different situation exists for orthotopic cornea transplants in mice. When allogeneic cornea grafts are placed in low-risk eyes, *only* donor-specific T cells of the 'indirect alloreactive' type can be detected [26, 27]. This is even the case when the donor cornea expresses foreign MHC class I and II antigens! (see table 2). When allogeneic corneas are grafted into high-risk recipient eyes, both 'direct' and 'indirect' alloreactive T cells are detected. Moreover, allogeneic cornea grafts placed in low-risk mouse eyes regularly induce the generation of donor-specific 'indirect' CD8$^+$ cytotoxic T cells, but not alloreactive T cells of the 'direct' type. In aggregate, the pattern of effector T cells elicited by orthotopic cornea transplants placed in low- and high-risk eyes indicates that the T-cell populations responsible for rejection of cornea transplants are likely to be primarily of the indirect alloreactive type, and therefore at least partially different from the T-cell populations that reject other types of solid organ transplants.

Immune Effector Modalities That Cause Rejection of Orthotopic Cornea Transplants in Laboratory Rodents

Acute rejection of orthotopic corneal transplants in mice occurs within 2–6 weeks of engraftment and is characterized by profound stromal opacity resulting from failure/loss of endothelial cells/function [24]. Numerous experiments indicate that donor-specific antibodies do not mediate rejection of this type. Instead, acute rejection of cornea transplants is mediated by CD4$^+$ T cells of the type that mediate delayed hypersensitivity [28, 29]. At the same time, there is no evidence that CD8$^+$ T cells mediate rejection of corneas; in fact, there is evidence that $CD8^+$ T cells are irrelevant to graft outcome early after keratoplasty (table 2) [30, 31]. The failure of $CD8^+$ T cells to participate in immune rejection of corneas stands in stark contrast to the situation for other types of solid tissue transplants.

The situation is made even more paradoxical by the facts that $CD8^+$ T cells recognize antigens of the MHC class I type, and that these types of antigens are the only MHC molecules expressed by corneal cells. By contrast, $CD4^+$ T cells recognize antigens of the MHC class II type, and these types of antigens are not expressed constitutively by corneal cells. Thus, a paradox emerges: corneal cells express class I MHC-encoded antigens but are not attacked by recipient $CD8^+$ T cells, and at the same time corneal cells express *no* class II MHC-encoded antigens, yet they are destroyed by recipient $CD4^+$ T cells. These data suggest that, especially for grafts placed in low-risk eyes, parenchymal cells of cornea grafts expressing disparate class I and II MHC antigens are largely invisible to 'direct' alloreactive T cells of the recipient.

In a sense this paradoxical situation serves as a suitable explanation for why MHC-encoded alloantigens on donor corneas, as detected by tissue typing, are likely to be of limited value in determining whether the graft will be rejected or not. But if that explanation contains truth, what explains the vulnerability to rejection of corneas that express minor H antigens?

Indirect Alloreactive T Cells and Self-MHC Bearing APCs

While the normal cornea used for grafting is essentially devoid of MHC class II-bearing dendritic cells of the Langerhans cell type, transplanted corneas rapidly acquire class II^+ cells of this type [31, 32]. To emphasize this point, treatment strategies designed to suppress migration of recipient dendritic cells and macrophages into the graft are quite successful at preventing or at least delaying cornea graft rejection [33]. In fact, the ability of an orthotopic corneal transplant to sensitize its recipient rests largely upon the capacity of recipient dendritic cells and macrophages to penetrate into the graft, especially the stroma.

Experimental evidence indicates that recipient dendritic cells function as APCs within the graft bed. These APCs first capture alloantigens released from dead and injured graft parenchymal cells, then they cleave the captured proteins into immunogenic peptides that are loaded onto the APCs' own MHC class I and II molecules. Subsequently, these recipient APCs enter lymphatics of the graft bed and carry their immunogenic signals to the draining (cervical) lymph nodes. At this site, naïve, recipient T cells – of the 'indirect alloreactive type' – are activated, differentiate into effector cells, and then disseminate systemically [34, 35].

As mentioned previously, both MHC and minor H antigens give rise to peptides that are recognized on self-MHC molecules by indirect alloreactive T cells. In most tissues, peptides derived from MHC class I and class II molecules are the predominant peptides found on APC MHC molecules. By contrast, in the cornea, where parenchymal cells express no MHC class II molecules, and reduced MHC class I molecules, minor H antigens from graft parenchymal cells are the major source of peptides displayed on self-MHC molecules expressed by infiltrating APCs. We believe, but have yet to prove, that preferential expression of minor H antigen-derived peptides (at the expense of MHC antigen-derived peptides) on infiltrating recipient APCs helps to explain why indirect alloreactive T cells with specificity for minor H antigens are the dominant effector cells found in mice receiving orthotopic corneal allografts that express both MHC and minor H antigens.

Indirect Alloreactive Effector T Cells and Rejection of Allogeneic Cornea Grafts in Low-Risk Eyes

Since MHC disparate corneal allografts placed in low-risk mouse eyes fail to activate direct alloreactive T cells, and since CD8$^+$ T cells have been found to be irrelevant to rejection of such grafts, the task of mediating graft rejection must rest solely with *CD4$^+$ T cells of the 'indirect' type* [24, 27, 28] (see table 2). The antigenic moieties recognized by these T cells are peptides derived from donor alloantigens that are displayed on self-MHC class II molecules. When graft donor and recipient share NO class II MHC molecules, then cells of the graft cannot serve as antigenic targets of indirect alloreactive CD4$^+$ T cells. Instead, infiltrating, recipient-derived APCs must serve this role. Consequently, when sensitized T cells enter the graft site, they recognize donor-derived antigens as peptides displayed by recipient APCs. Recognition leads to T-cell activation and the release of a range of cytokines (especially IFN-γ and TNF-α) that recruit to the site non-specific immune effectors such as macrophages and neutrophils, and these cells in turn mediate delayed hypersensitivity. Thus, rejection of the cornea occurs because of the toxicity of non-specific inflammatory mediators, rather than because effector T cells have killed corneal cells directly. In a very real sense, the cornea 'dies' as an innocent bystander to the intense, destructive immune inflammation that is triggered in its microenvironment by T cells responding to donor antigens on recipient APCs.

When donor and recipient of grafts placed in low-risk eyes share one or more class II MHC alloantigens, the situation changes. During cornea graft rejection, endothelial cells of the graft begin to express class II MHC molecules, and recent experiments indicate that these molecules are expressed without the invariant chain, Ii, i.e. in the absence of the class II transactivator (CIITA) [36]. Under normal circumstances, class II molecules are co-synthesized with Ii because both genes are under the control of CIITA [37]. Ii molecules complex with newly synthesized class II molecules in the endoplasmic reticulum, and thereby prevent endogenous peptides from occupying the groove on class II molecules until they reach the endosomal compartments. Enzymes in endo-somes eventually cleave Ii away, permitting peptides from this compartment to be loaded onto class II MHC molecules. In this manner, class II MHC molecules normally display peptides derived from exogenous sources (foreign antigens). However, expression of class II MHC molecules by corneal endothelium occurs in the absence of Ii, and this allows endogenous peptides to access the class II groove. This is particularly relevant because minor H antigens are largely intracellular (endogenous), not surface, molecules, and their recognition by T cells requires that their peptides be loaded onto MHC molecules. Thus, during corneal allograft rejection, class II MHC molecules are expressed on endothelial cells by a CIITA-independent process, and as a consequence of the failure of Ii expression, these class II molecules display intracellular peptides that are largely derived from minor H antigens.

The foregoing discussion, though complex and detailed, helps to explain why a corneal allograft that shares at least one MHC class II molecule with its recipient is especially vulnerable to immune rejection. In such grafts, two targets of invading T cells emerge: recipient APCs and donor endothelium. Both cell types express MHC class II molecules that the T cells recognize as 'self', and both cell types display minor H peptides on these MHC class II molecules. We have obtained recent evidence that this situation enhances the vulnerability of corneal grafts to immune rejection [38]. BALB.B and C57BL/6 mice possess the same MHC alleles, but differ at multiple minor H loci. We found that BALB.B mice reject 25% of corneas donated by C57BL/6 mice in which the class II gene is inactivated (grafts cannot express class II molecules). BALB.B mice reject 50% of corneas donated by C57BL/6 mice in whom the CIITA gene is inactivated (grafts can still express class II molecules by a CIITA-independent process), and this incidence of graft rejection is identical to that of BALB.B mice that receive cornea grafts from normal C57BL/6 mice. Thus, when donor and recipient share one or more class II MHC alleles, parenchymal cells of the graft serve as targets of T-cell activation. Together with infiltrating recipient APCs, corneal parenchymal cells increase the vulnerability of the graft to rejection, primarily because in this circumstance parenchymal cells of the graft (epithelium, keratocytes, endothelium) are now capable of expressing MHC class II molecules.

Direct and Indirect Alloreactive Effector T Cells and Rejection of Allogeneic Cornea Grafts in High-Risk Eyes

The incidence of cornea graft rejection is markedly increased in mice when grafts are placed in neovascularized and inflamed graft beds [39]. Because these grafts elicit both 'direct' and 'indirect' alloreactive T cells (see table 2), and because these graft beds manifestly lack the property of immune privilege [32], one would anticipate that allogeneic class I and class II MHC molecules on the graft would serve readily as targets of attacking T cells. By this logic, tissue matching of donor and recipient in humans for MHC antigens would be predicted to reduce the incidence of graft rejection in high-risk eyes. Yet, it remains controversial that this is the case [13–16, and other chapters in this book]. It is worth inquiring what has been learned from the murine experimental system that might shed light on this paradox.

The peculiar resistance of murine corneal allografts to rejection by direct alloreactive CD8$^+$ T cells is a case in point. BALB/c mice that have received MHC plus minor H disparate cornea grafts from C57BL/6 donors are largely prevented from rejecting their grafts if their CD4$^+$ T cells are eliminated [40]. Since these mice contain easily detectable direct alloreactive CD8$^+$ T cells that are cytotoxic for appropriate target cells in vitro [27, 28, 41] there is clearly something about the cornea that prevents cytotoxic T cells from destroying the graft. Part of the 'something' may be inherent resistance to immune cytotoxicity. First, corneal endothelial cells constitutively express CD95 ligand (CD95L), a receptor that binds CD95, a molecule expressed on the surface of activated CD95$^+$ T cells [42]. When engaged by CD95L$^+$ target cells in this manner, CD95$^+$ T cells are unable to carry out their effector functions, and, instead, they undergo programmed cell death. Perhaps this is one reason why CD8$^+$ T cells of the direct alloreactive type fail to destroy the endothelial cells of cornea grafts bearing class I alloantigens that they express. Experiments in mice indicate that CD95 ligand expression on orthotopic corneal allografts prevents these grafts from rejection [43, 44]. Second, corneal endothelial cells display inherent resistance to lysis by cytotoxic T cells, resistance that is even present when the endothelial cells are derived from mice without functional CD95 ligand molecules. Experiments conducted by Haskova et al. [45] have demonstrated that corneal endothelial cells, even cells stimulated with IFN-γ, fail to be lysed in vitro when exposed to specifically primed cytotoxic T cells. Perhaps for these reasons, or for reasons yet to be defined, CD8$^+$ T cells play no role in acute rejection of corneal allografts in high-risk eyes [27, 28, 41]. It is therefore not surprising that tissue matching for class I alloantigens in humans has largely failed to improve the fate of corneal transplants, whether placed in low- or high-risk eyes.

In murine high-risk eyes, CD4$^+$ T cells alone mediate rejection of orthotopic corneal transplants, and both direct and indirect alloreactive T cells contribute to rejection [22]. A prediction from these results would be that tissue typing and matching of donors and recipients for class II MHC antigens should improve the success rate of penetrating keratoplasties. Yet, it remains controversial whether tissue matching of this type actually improves graft outcome, and the reasons for this situation are by no means obvious. In the mouse model system, minor H antigens continue to be stronger barriers than MHC antigens to graft acceptance when donor corneas are placed in high-risk eyes. But if direct alloreactive, donor class II-specific CD4$^+$ T cells were primarily responsible for graft rejection in high-risk eyes, minor H antigens should prove to be *less* important. It would appear that MHC molecules on parenchymal cells of cornea grafts are surprisingly ineffective at serving as targets for attacking T cells.

Immune Privilege and the Fate of Penetrating Keratoplasty

The existence of immune privilege in the anterior chamber of the eye influences the fate of corneal grafts since these grafts form the anterior wall of the chamber [46, 47]. Moreover, immune privilege is a constitutive feature of the cornea itself as a tissue [48]. It is likely that the combination of anterior chamber immune privilege with cornea immune privilege confounds our ability to understand the reasons why cornea transplants sometimes succeed and sometimes fail. Experimental strategies that abolish immune privilege in the anterior chamber of mouse eyes significantly increase the incidence and vigor of rejection of orthotopic corneal transplants [39]. Similarly, experimental strategies that alter the cornea graft itself (for example, by equipping the cornea with activated APCs of donor origin) markedly enhance the vulnerability of the graft to immune rejection [31, 32]. Finally, in mice that accept their orthotopic corneal allografts, anterior chamber associated immune deviation (ACAID) arises within 6–8 weeks [49]. There is evidence that the long-term survival of these grafts is predicated on the persistence of donor-specific ACAID. Thus, it is possible factors that impose immune privilege (ACAID) on the anterior chamber and the cornea may act to shift the antigenic burden of the graft from MHC-encoded alloantigens to the antigens encoded by minor H genes.

The inability of IFN-γ-stimulated corneal endothelium to activate the CIITA gene (described above) may be an example of such a factor. Other immune privileged sites such as placenta and brain appear to have a similar prohibition against expression of CIITA [50–52]. Similarly, constitutive CD95 ligand expression is a feature that the cornea shares with other immune privileged sites, such as the testis [53]. Ferguson and colleagues [54] believe that

CD95 ligand expression in the eye is an essential component of the process by which eye-derived antigens induce ACAID, a conclusion also reached from research results in our laboratory [55]. Immune privilege may act to reduce the importance of MHC antigens in transplantation, thereby unmasking the potential of minor H antigens to promote graft rejection.

Minor H Antigens and Failed Penetrating Keratoplasty in Humans

If there are similarities between mouse and human with respect to corneal transplantation immunobiology, then minor H antigens may be very important for corneal graft rejection in the clinic. Circumstantial evidence already exists to suggest that this is the case. In the Collaborative Corneal Transplantation Study (CCTS) that evaluated the influence of HLA- and ABO-encoded antigens on the fate of human corneas grafted into high-risk eyes, grafts mismatched for ABO antigens showed statistically significant vulnerability to rejection compared to ABO-matched grafts [14]. While antibodies against the A&B isohemagglutinins are important in blood typing, these antibodies play little or no role in cornea transplant rejection. Instead, the polymorphic enzymes (glycosyltransferases) that create the A and the B antigens from the O antigen may serve as minor H antigens. We have speculated that peptides derived from the glycosyltransferase that creates the A substance (in type A individuals) can be loaded onto class II molecules and serve as targets of primed CD4$^+$ T cells – just as any minor H antigen might do [14]. Perhaps type O or type B individuals that receive a cornea from a type A donor acquire primed CD4$^+$ T cells that recognize peptides derived from the type A glycosyltransferase in the context of 'self' class II MHC molecules. Experience with murine transplants suggests that rejection of the graft should be the outcome. The experiments described above [23, 45] already demonstrate that a single minor H antigen disparity can be sufficient to cause irreversible cornea graft rejection in mice. Thus, the vulnerability of ABO mismatched cornea transplants to rejection may presage the importance of minor H antigen disparity in human penetrating keratoplasty.

In summary, in the mouse model system, minor H antigens are significantly more important to the outcome of orthotopic corneal grafts than are antigens encoded by MHC class I and II genes. The reasons for this unusual feature of the cornea as a graft include (a) lack of MHC class II expression on any cells of the normal cornea, including dendritic cells and macrophages of bone marrow origin; (b) expression of MHC class II molecules on corneal endothelial cells during rejection via a CIITA-independent pathway that favors the loading of minor H antigen-derived peptides on self class II molecules; (c) recipient APCs that infiltrate the graft and display peptides derived from donor alloantigens on their self class II molecules; (d) reduced MHC class I expression on corneal parenchymal cells, especially corneal endothelium; (e) preferential loading of peptides derived from minor H, rather than MHC, antigens on MHC class II molecules on recipient APCs because MHC expression on corneal cells is much reduced; (f) resistance of corneal endothelium to lysis by both direct and indirect alloreactive CD8$^+$ T cells, and (g) immune privilege that preferentially inhibits rejection by direct alloreactive T cells specific for MHC-encoded class I and II antigens.

If a similar situation applies to humans, then much needs to be done to identify minor H antigens on human tissues [56], and to develop strategies for matching donors and recipients for these antigens. Although this is a difficult area of research, the rewards are likely to be significant – as has begun to be the case for minor H antigen research in other types of solid organ transplants in humans.

Acknowledgement

Research reported in this communication has been supported by grant EY 10765 from the National Eye Institute, USA.

References

1   Medawar PB: Immunity to homologous grafted skin. III. The fate of skin homografts transplanted to the brain, to subcutaneous tissue, and to the anterior chamber of the eye. Br J Exp Pathol 1948;29:58–69.
2   Autoimmunity and Transplantation; in Janeway CA, Travers P, Walport M, Shlomchik MJ (eds): Immunobiology. London, Current Biology Ltd, 2001, pp 501–552.
3   Opelz G: Factors influencing long-term graft loss. The Collaborative Transplant Study. Transplant Proc 2000;32:647–649.
4   Whitsett CF, Stulting RD: The distribution of HLA antigens on human corneal tissue. Invest Ophthalmol Vis Sci 1984;25:519–524.
5   Pepose JS, Gardner KM, Nestor MS, Foos RY, Pettit TH: Detection of HLA class I and II antigens in rejected human corneal allografts. Ophthalmology 1985;92:1480–1484.
6   Treseler PA, Sanfilippo F: The expression of major histocompatibility complex and leukocyte antigens by cells in the rat cornea. Transplantation 1986;41:248–252.
7   Wang HM, Kaplan HJ, Chan WC, Johnson M: The distribution and ontogeny of MHC antigens in murine ocular tissue. Invest Ophthalmol Vis Sci 1987;28:1383–1389.
8   Streilein JW, Toews GB, Bergstresser PR: Corneal allografts fail to express Ia antigens. Nature 1979;282:326–327.
9   Volker-Dieben HJM, Kok-van A, Alphen CC, Lansbergen Q, Persign GG: Different influences on corneal graft survival in 539 transplants. Acta Ophthalmol 1982;60:190–202.
10 Ehlers N, Ahrons S: Corneal transplantation and histocompatibility. Acta Ophthalmol 1971; 49:513–527.
11 Batchelor JS, Casey TA, Givvs DC, Prasad SS, Lloyd DF, James A: HLA matching and corneal grafting. Lancet 1976;i: 551–554.
12 Stark WJ, Taylor HR, Bias WB, Maumenee AE: Histocompatibility (HLA) antigens and keratoplasty. Am J Ophthalmol 1978;86:596–604.

13 Völker-Dieben HJ, Claas FH, Schreuder GM, Schipper RF, Pels E, Persijn GG, Smits J, D'Amaro J: Beneficial effect of HLA-DR matching on the survival of corneal allografts. Transplantation 2000;70:640–648.

14 The Collaborative Corneal Transplantation Studies Research Group: The Collaborative Corneal Transplantation Studies (CCTS). Effectiveness of histocompatibility matching in high-risk corneal transplantation. Arch Ophthalmol 1992;110:1392–1403.

15 Vail A, Gore SM, Bradley BA, et al: Influence of donor and histocompatibility factors on corneal graft outcome. Transplantation 1994;58:1210–1216.

16 Gore SM, Vail A, Bradley BA, et al: HLA-DR matching in corneal transplantation. Systemic review of published evidence. Transplantation 1995;60:1033–1039.

17 Williams KA, Coster DJ: Penetrating corneal transplantation in the inbred rat: A new model. Invest Ophthalmol Vis Sci 1985;26:23–30.

18 Sonoda Y, Streilein JW: Orthotopic corneal transplantation in mice – Evidence that the immunogenic rules of rejection do not apply. Transplantation. 1992;54:694–704.

19 Joo CK, Pepose JS, Stuart PM: T cell mediated responses in a murine model of orthotopic corneal transplantation. Invest Ophthalmol Vis Sci 1995;36:1530–1540.

20 Sano Y, Ksander BR, Streilein JW: Minor H, rather than MHC, alloantigens offer the greater barrier to successful orthotopic corneal transplantation in mice. Transplant Immunol 1996;4:53–56.

21 Yamada J, Streilein JW: Fate of orthotopic corneal allografts in C57BL/6 mice. Transplant Immunol 1998;6:161–168.

22 Sano Y, Ksander BR, Streilein JW: Murine orthotopic corneal transplantation in 'high-risk' eyes. Rejection is dictated primarily by weak rather than strong alloantigens. Invest Ophthalmol Vis Sci 1997;38:1130–1138.

23 Haskova Z, Roopenian DC, Ksander BR: An immunodominant minor histocompatibility alloantigen that terminates immune privilege and initiates corneal graft rejection. Invest Ophthalmol Vis Sci (in press).

24 Streilein JW: Regional immunity and ocular immune privilege; in Streilein JW (ed): Chemical Immunology, vol 73: Immune Response and the Eye. Basel, Karger, 1999, pp 11–38.

25 Niederkorn JY: The immune privilege of corneal allografts. Transplantation 1999;67:1503–1508.

26 Shoskes DA, Wood KJ: Indirect presentation of MHC antigens in transplantation. Immunol Today 1994;13:32–38.

27 Ksander B, Sano Y, Streilein JW: Role of donor-specific cytotoxic T cells in rejection of corneal allografts in normal and high-risk eyes. Transplant Immunol 1996;4:49–51.

28 Yamada J, Kurimoto I, Streilein JW: Role of CD4+ T cells in immunobiology of orthotopic corneal transplants in mice. Invest Ophthalmol Vis Sci 1999;40:2614–2621.

29 Sonoda Y, Sano Y, Ksander B, Streilein JW: Characterization of cell-mediated immune responses elicited by orthotopic corneal allografts in mice. Invest Ophthalmol Vis Sci 1995;36:427–434.

30 Yamada J, Ksander BR, Streilein JW: Cytotoxic T cells play no essential role in acute rejection of orthotopic corneal allografts in mice. Invest Ophthalmol Vis Sci 2001;42:386–392.

31 Peeler JS, Niederkorn JY: Antigen presentation by Langerhans cells in vivo: Donor derived Ia+ Langerhans cells are required for induction of delayed type hypersensitivity but not for cytotoxic T lymphocyte responses to alloantigens. J Immunol 1986;136:4362–4371.

32 Sano Y, Ksander BR, Streilein JW: Langerhans cells, orthotopic corneal allografts, and direct and indirect pathways of T cell allorecognition. Invest Ophthal Vis Sci 2000;41:1422–1431.

33 Mohomad-Reza D, Yamada J, Streilein JW: Topical IL-1 receptor antagonist promotes corneal transplant survival. Transplantation 1997;63:1501–1507.

34 Yamagami S, Mohomad-Reza D: The critical role of lymph nodes in corneal alloimmunization and graft rejection. Invest Ophthalmol Vis Sci 2001;42:1293–1298.

35 Boisgerault F, Liu T, Anosova N, Ehrlich E, Dana MR, Benichou G: Role of CD4+ and CD8+ T cells in allorecognition: Lessons from corneal transplantation. J Immunol 2001;167:1891–1899.

36 Arancibia CV, George AJT, Ono SJ, Streilein JW: Expression of CIITA reconstitutes class II MHC expression on corneal endothelial cells: Implications for antigen presentation. Invest Ophthalmol Vis Sci 2001;42:S471.

37 Harton JA, Ting JPY: Class II transactivator: Mastering the art of major histocompatibility complex expression. Mol Cell Biol 2000;20:6185–6194.

38 Osawa H, Arancibia CV, Ting JPY, Streilein JW: Self class II MHC molecules carrying donor-derived peptides are the primary, while donor MHC molecules are only secondary, targets of the CD4[+] T cells that reject orthotopic corneal allografts. Invest Ophthal Vis Sci 2001;42:S471.

39 Sano Y, Ksander BR, Streilein JW: Fate of orthotopic corneal allografts in eyes that cannot support anterior chamber-associated immune deviation induction. Invest Ophthalmol Vis Sci 1995;36: 2176–2185.

40 He YG, Ross J, Niederkorn JY: Promotion of murine orthotopic corneal allograft survival by systemic administration of anti-CD4 monoclonal antibody. Invest Ophthalmol Vis Sci 1991;32: 2723–2728.

41 Hegde S, Niederkorn JY: The role of cytotoxic T lymphocytes in corneal allograft rejection. Invest Ophthalmol Vis Sci 2000;41:3341–3347.

42 Griffith TS, Brunner T, Fletcher S, Green D, Ferguson T: Fas ligand-induced apoptosis as a mechanism of immune privilege. Science 1995;270:1189–1192.

43 Stuart PM, Griffith TS, Usui N, Pepose J, Yu X, Ferguson TA: CD95 ligand (FasL)-induced apoptosis is necessary for corneal allograft survival. J Clin Invest 1997;99:396–402.

44 Yamagami S, Kawashima H, Tsuru T, Yamagami H, Kayagaki N, Yagita H, Gregerson DS: Role of Fas-Fas ligand interactions in the immunorejection of allogeneic mouse corneal transplants. Transplantation 1997;64:1107–1111.

45 Haskova Z, Arancibia CV, Christianson GJ, Roopenian DC, Ksander BR: Altered proteasome expression in corneal endothelial cells contributes to immune privilege (abstract). Invest Ophthalmol Vis Sci 2001;42:2539.

46 Yamada J, Streilein JW: Induction of anterior chamber-associated immune deviation by corneal allografts placed in the anterior chamber. Invest Ophthalmol Vis Sci 1997;38:2833–2843.

47 Streilein JW, Ksander BR, Taylor AW: Immune deviation in relation to ocular immune privilege. J Immunol 1997;158:3557–3560.

48 Hori J, Joyce N, Streilein JW: Epithelium-deficient corneal allografts display immune privilege beneath the kidney capsule. Invest Ophthalmol Vis Sci 2000;41:443–452.

49 Sonoda Y, Streilein JW: Impaired cell-mediated immunity in mice bearing healthy orthotopic corneal allografts. J Immunol 1993;150:1727–1734.

50 Butterworth B, Khong T, Loke Y, Robertson W: Human cytotrophoblast populations studied by monoclonal antibodies using single and double biotin-avidin-peroxidase immunocytochemistry. J Histochem Cytochem 1985;33:977–983.

51 Borthwick G, Holmes R, Stirrat G: Abnormal expression of class II MHC antigens in placentae from patients with pemphigoid gestationis: Analysis of class II MHC subregion product expression. Placenta 1988;9:81–94.

52 Armstrong TD, Clements VK, Martin BK, Ting JPY, Ostrand-Rosenberg S: Major histocompatibility complex class II-transfected tumor cells present endogenous antigen and are potent inducers of tumor-specific immunity. Proc Natl Acad Sci USA 1997;94:6888–6891.

53 Bellgrau D, Gold D, Selawry H, Moore J, Franzusoff A, Duke RC: A role for CD95 ligand in preventing graft rejection. Nature 1995;377:630–632.

54 Griffith TS, Yu X, Herndon JM, Green DR, Ferguson TA: CD95-induced apoptosis of lymphocytes in an immune privileged site induces immunological tolerance. Immunity 1996;5:7–16.

55 Kezuka T, Streilein JW: Evidence for multiple CD95–CD95 ligand interactions in anterior chamber associated immune deviation (ACAID) induced by soluble protein antigen. Immunology 2000;99: 451–457.

56 Goulmy E: Minor histocompatibility antigens: From T cell recognition to peptide identification (editorial). Hum Immunol 1997;54:8–14.

J. Wayne Streilein, MD
Schepens Eye Research Institute,
20 Staniford St., Boston, MA 02114 (USA)
Tel. +1 617 9127422, Fax +1 617 9120115, E-Mail waynes@vision.eri.harvard.edu

Sundmacher R (ed): Adequate HLA Matching in Keratoplasty.
Dev Ophthalmol. Basel, Karger, 2003, vol 36, pp 89–97

....

A Clinician's Outlook on HLA Matching for Keratoplasty

Rainer Sundmacher

Universität Düsseldorf, Klinik für Augenheilkunde, Düsseldorf, Deutschland

Abstract

Background: A clinician's view of HLA matching for keratoplasty (kp) must basically be a rather pragmatic one: as immunosuppressives are getting more and more potent with acceptable toxicity, what advantage does HLA matching offer in addition to or supplementing immunosuppressives? Also, one wants to know what can be expected of further fundamental progress in this field in the future.

Methods: The author tries to answer these questions based on three sources: (1) the papers in this volume, all written by highly experienced and leading specialists in their field; (2) the international kp literature, and (3) the author's own kp experiences of 30 years' duration with many clinical studies derived therefrom.

Results: There is no doubt that HLA matching has a great potential in kp and works already well on a statistical basis in high-risk as well as in normal-risk patients. In the individual kp patient, however, a decision as to what extent current HLA matching would be useful and advisable is a question far less easy to answer. This is exemplified by clinical examples.

Conclusions: HLA matching, as it is practically feasible now, is recommended as an adjunctive immunoprophylactic measure for every patient for whom the calculable waiting time is tolerable. Matching should, whenever possible, comprise HLA-A/-B as well as -DR matching and should, if possible, be performed on solid molecular grounds. In the future, the new 'weighted' concept of permissible versus taboo mismatches will become more and more operative and will substitute the current still simple matching criteria which can nothing more than respect unweighted numbers of fitting alleles. It seems probable that sometime later still more refined systems (e.g. 'minors') will supplement or even partially substitute current HLA typing. In whichever direction typing and matching will continue to develop in the future, it seems clear by now that a systematic start into typing and matching in keratoplasty is inevitable for all those surgeons and cornea bankers who want to keep on with progress in this field.

The symposium on recent developments in the field of HLA matching for penetrating keratoplasty at the Annual Meeting of the German Ophthalmological Society in Berlin, 2001, was held in an attempt to bring together the newest clinical and basic immunologic aspects which might be relevant for a reappraisal of the clinical value of HLA matching.

A reappraisal of HLA matching for keratoplasty has become necessary because the results of a number of recent clinical studies have once more proven that HLA matching does have a significant effect on clear survival of corneal grafts. This is in contrast to the results of several older studies, which are still often cited. Other reasons which call for a reappraisal are the many new and sometimes conflicting results and aspects which clinical and experimental immunologists have contributed to the immunology of keratoplasty during the last years.

As the results of scientific studies will often be conflicting, but as there can, of course, be only one medical truth, it follows that time has come for a decision whether or not HLA matching is of clinical significance in keratoplasty in humans and therefore whether it should be applied. As a clinician I answer this question without hesitation by yes. This yes, however, is not expressed without limitations. I certainly do not believe that currently available HLA matching will solve all or the majority of the immunologic problems associated with penetrating keratoplasty. The best we can say at present is that HLA matching already is and probably will become even more in the future a valuable adjunct to other measures which are suitable to reduce immune complications after penetrating keratoplasty in man. It is necessary, therefore, that we take proper advantage of these chances and care about this field much more intensively than we have done in the past. Let us look at various aspects step by step:

Medical Therapy by Immune-Suppressive/Immune-Modulating Agents Will Stay the Most Important Measure to Enhance Corneal Transplant Survival

There is no doubt that medical immune therapy – short-term topical steroids for the easy cases up to potentially dangerous systemic long-term application of cyclosporin A, mycophenolate mofetil and similar drugs for high-risk cases – will stay the most important measure to enhance corneal transplant survival. Alternative or adjunctive immunologic therapy, however, is urgently needed in addition for all cases in which such medical therapy is not applicable – which is not a rare event. Further, one should generally strive to reduce the immunologic stimuli by the graft most effectively in order to spare as much of these drugs as possible. This will not only reduce the threat of severe side effects and complications but also enlarge the chances for a longer graft survival. If such an adjuvant immunologic measure has been proven effective and harmless, then it should be most welcome. It is my conviction that HLA matching is such a measure.

HLA Matching Is the Currently Only Available Effective Measure to Support Medical Immune Therapy

The results of the clinical studies presented in this volume prove unanimously that HLA matching is an effective adjunct to basic medical immune therapy. This means, vice versa, that the older studies, which could not show such a result, were wrong in this respect. I do not want to repeat here again all the arguments which speak against those studies. If the reader still has any doubts, then he should go back to the original articles and study these carefully again, especially all the items that have been criticized.

I would also like to avoid a discussion of the often put question what part of the MHC in man is the most important one for matching the HLA-A/-B or -DR loci, because this question is probably too simple and does not help much in the long run. From the clinical studies on which we rely here, it can be deducted that there must be relevant alleles in each of these subsystems, otherwise it could not be explained why fairly good matched HLA-A/-B alleles and good matched -DR alleles both lead to significant positive results. As Reinhard et al. have shown that in normal-risk patients a matching of only either -A/-B or -DR gave sub-significant results whereas the joined typing and matching of all 6 alleles (4 from HLA-A/-B, and 2 from -DR) delivered significant results, it seems probable that the joined matching of -A/-B plus -DR can be currently regarded to be the optimal clinical approach. For low-risk patients such a joint matching is necessary to reach statistical significance. High-risk patients reach this level already by matching one of the two subsystems. But it is certainly no mistake to match all 6 alleles also in these patients, if this is possible logistically. If only matching in the -A/-B subsystem is logistically feasible, then the split alleles should be used instead of the broad ones in order to safely reach statistical significance as Beekhuis et al. have shown.

At this point I would like to address a basic problem with current matching: The clinical significance of HLA matching has been shown only for patient *groups*, i.e. an individual patient will benefit from a 'good' match only with a certain probability. But it may also be that he will not benefit at all! Claas has explained in his article the reason for this: Every allele of recipient and donor may have a very different importance, and this importance is not absolute but changes with the allele configuration of recipient and donor. Both also act on one another. It may be, therefore, that a 'bad' match (e.g. 3/6) in one pairing is immunologically more beneficial than a 'good' match (5/6) in another pairing. As we barely have information up to now about the differential importance of HLA alleles in different constellations, we cannot yet select for this criterion but must be content with selecting the highest graded match possible for an individual patient, because this statistically – but not invariably – gives us the best chances for a success.

The matching grades, which must be required, are at least 2 out of 4 in HLA-A/-B, or 2 out of 2 in HLA-DR for high-risk patients. For low-risk patients it should be at least 4 out of 6, both subsystems taken together.

At the end of this paragraph I would like to specifically acknowledge the important work of Henny Völker-Dieben. Her work has so often and so vigorously been criticized and attacked in the past, that others would presumably have long given up. Henny did not, and what she has presented to us in the end may really be called a milestone in clinical immunology of keratoplasty. Thank you!

HLA Matching Is Not Always Possible and Not Even Always Advisable for Various Reasons. The Decision For or Against a Matched Graft Remains an Individual One

As the logistic possibilities for HLA matching are very different at various sites, I will restrict myself in this paragraph to describing how we make our decisions pro or contra a matched graft in Düsseldorf: We start with a complete typing of every recipient, normal- and high-risk. Then we calculate the probability within which waiting time we can offer to this patient from our own cornea bank (and from Bioimplant Service, Leiden, The Netherlands) a 'perfect' graft (6/6), a 'good' graft (5/6) or a 'fairly good' graft (4/6) [see Böhringer's article, this volume]. On the basis of this logistic background information, the clinical situation of the patient determines our pro or contra. Because of the multitude of individual aspects, it makes no great sense to formulate specific rules. I describe, instead, as examples, some constellations which are frequent:

(a) For a 75-year-old lady with Fuchs' dystrophy I would advise a random graft, because in this normal risk case the chances are good that the graft with topical steroid therapy will keep clear as long as the patient lives. If the chances for a 5/6 match are excellent, however (e.g. only 4 months' waiting time), then I would advise her to wait for this chance. Such a relatively short waiting period is also acceptable for old patients. It is in fact shorter than the waiting time on most lists for random grafts all over the world.

(b) For a 50-year-old car driver with traumatic corneal scarring and impending unemployment I would strongly recommend a random procedure unless a well-matched graft is accidentally at hand. This patient needs professional rehabilitation as quickly as possible, which is most important for him socially. Waiting, and be it only for months, might enhance his problems enormously without guarantee that waiting time pays off later in terms of longer graft survival.

(c) If a 35-year-old teacher with monolateral severe keratoconus states that he can still manage in his profession and that above all he is basically concerned about how long the new cornea will last in his eye, I would strongly recommend the best matched graft that we possibly can get for him. Which matching grade is achievable for him in which time will be told by the Böhringer formula. What waiting time this patient regards as reasonable has to be determined by himself. In case he has very rare alleles that waiting time for him will be very long even for a 4/6 match, then he would be advised that a random graft is the only possible way and insured that such a random graft is not necessarily worse than a matched graft and may function well over a long period of time.

(d) In a 3-year-old child with monolateral severe corneal laceration 6 months ago and beginning strabismus, I would not wait for any matched graft but operate as quickly as possible with a random graft in order to fight amblyopia. It is of prime importance here to have a well-functioning graft for the next couple of years. It should mostly be possible to accomplish this goal with a random cornea. If this emergency graft should gradually fail some years later, then, of course, there is no longer time pressure, and then this child or youngster should be given the opportunity for a matched (second) graft.

(e) In every case of high-risk keratoplasty, which is scheduled for a long systemic immune therapy, I would strongly recommend waiting for the best available matched graft. Which matching grade is achievable, again, depends on the recipient's alleles.

(f) The only general statement which I would like to make at the end of this paragraph is that every patient in our clinic is given the opportunity – if ever possible – to decide for himself after information about the medical background and the consequences whether or not he accepts the waiting time for a matched graft and for what matching grade.

Before HLA-Matched Grafts Can Be Efficiently Offered on a Larger Scale, Adequate Logistic Facilities Have to Be Organized

This is a difficult topic, especially because some money may be involved. I might state, however, that from my personal experience, with the help of engaged organizations (e.g. Lions Cornea Bank in our case) and with pertinent pressure on all responsible persons in the administrations, things are achievable which for decades have been said to be 'impossible'. All is possible in this field, if we do want it. The German Federal Medical Council (Bundesärztekammer) has for example written in its guidelines for cornea banks that HLA matching should be applied whenever this is regarded state of the art. This obliges the cornea banks to deliver matched grafts. Delivery (matching) can only be optimal if there is a maximally large list of recipients on one side, which can be matched with a maximally large list of available typed grafts on the other side. The latter, of course, is optimally achievable only by virtually typing *all* corneal grafts. Again, most people would say 'impossible'! Come to our cornea bank and see – it's possible! It has been made possible by the introduction of molecular typing techniques which are not only by far more precise than the serological methods, it is also important that they can be performed from any tiny bit of tissue, e.g. from a part of the donor's scleral rim [see Doxiadis, this volume].

Our vision is that as many cornea banks as possible in every country build up such facilities and join in a network for allocation of matched corneas. These national networks may further interact internationally, which would enormously enlarge the chances for a matched graft even for patients with rare alleles. This is the vision, but tiny first steps have already been made also in this field, e.g. by a matching collaboration between our own local cornea bank and Bioimplant Services, Leiden, which currently affords about the largest amount of typed corneas in Central Europe and allocates them internationally [see de By, this volume].

A further matter of importance is the way in which donor corneas are preserved. Cornea banks all over the world currently mostly use short-term preservation techniques, which allow for about 7 days on an average from taking the cornea from the donor until suturing it into the recipient. In this limited time period, however, much more laboratory and organizational work has to be done when switching from random to matched graft allocation. From our experience there might arise organizational difficulties simply from lack of time with the short-term preservation methods, especially if the corneas have to be shipped over quite a distance. This lack of time does not exist if a bank works with long-time cultivation methods, which currently give us up to 4 weeks to accomplish all the additional tasks associated with typing and matching. It should be easier, more secure and more successful, therefore, to allocate matched corneas nationwide and internationally, if a bank uses long-term cultivation, which already is by far the most frequent type in Central Europe. Short-term preservation banks may, of course, also be successful in managing these time problems, but they will have to struggle much more.

Current HLA Matching Is Only the Start into a More Efficient Induction of Tolerance in the Future

It is beyond the scope of these short practical notes to elaborate and comment on the many fascinating aspects of current research in the vast field of transplantation immunology. As we discussed, for example, at the Symposium on Soluble MHC, Immunoregulation and Tolerance in Transplantation, held in Regensburg, Germany, March 2002. It is probable that one or the other of these projects will reach clinical significance in the future and then provide us with a far more differentiated armamentarium for induction of tolerance than available nowadays with matching alone.

Matching will be much improved and made much more efficient if the concept of permissible and taboo HLA mismatches [see Claas, this volume] will have been worked out in such a way that it is applicable on a broad and efficient basis for daily immunological practice. As already mentioned above, this concept tries to exploit the fact that the different HLA alleles evidently have very different importance in terms of influencing tolerance depending on whether they are of donor or recipient origin and also dependent on the whole set of alleles which may influence one another – a complex but very promising project.

Claas has also been working on another project (HLA matchmaker), that at first glance does not seem to be related to problems with keratoplasty: influencing chronic immune reactions by avoiding alloantibody formation. Up to now, we have identified in keratoplasty only a clinically well-defined chronic endothelial cellular immune reaction with characteristic endotheliitic precipitates. This type of chronic immune reaction is easily influenced by long-term, low-dose topical steroids. There seems to be no need, therefore, for more action in this field. There is another phenomenon, however, which I suspect also to be of immunologic pathophysiology although neither immune cells nor any other clinically evident inflammation has ever been clinically detected: chronic idiopathic endothelial cell loss in the graft. This cell loss is so severe over the years that it limits the ultimate life span of practically every graft. Consequently, corneal transplants do normally not survive longer than some 15 or 20 years at the most, even if a classical (cellular) immune reaction has never been detected. It has been my hypothesis for many years – still unproven – that some very slow, subclinical alloantibody action causes this chronic loss phenomenon. If this is true, Claas' matchmaker project may also be pertinent for keratoplasty patients and help to expand the ultimate life span of grafts beyond their current limits. This would be most important for every patient under 60 years, i.e. for most patients.

The excellent and highly interesting article of Streilein in this volume puts forward two aspects which at first glance seem to deviate from what had been presented before by others. At second glance, the differences are little.

Streilein believes, according to his vast experiences with a multitude of animal experiments for studying the various aspects of immunologic privilege of the anterior chamber and the cornea, that HLA matching cannot be expected to bring about much success in keratoplasty. This skepticism, nota bene, concerns only keratoplasty because of the special immunologic conditions of the eye, it does not concern other transplantations. I have no difficulties in basically agreeing. My clinical judgement also has told me that HLA matching, as currently possible, is by no means a very potent action – although in selected patients it may well be! But one cannot deny that on average it has a significant adjunctive immunologic influence and should therefore consequently be applied. Only with consequent and broad application of typing and matching techniques will we be able to sample more and more valid clinical data which will enable us to further systematically improve this method. This aspect, that we have been and will be dependent on broad-based clinical studies, has mostly been overlooked, and broad-based help has not been at hand until now. Putting it in a picture, I would say that Streilein, as a basic scientist, clearly sees where the deficits of current HLA matching still are. Accordingly, for him 'the glass is half empty'. I am, however, as a clinician, more than happy with and thankful for any clinical progress. For me, therefore, 'the glass is half full'.

Finally, Streilein is convinced from his keratoplasty studies in mice that the MHC plays less a role for tolerance induction in keratoplasty than the so-called 'minors', a currently largely expanding new research area in transplantation immunology. He postulates that also in man, 'minors' may be more important than the HLA system. That may, of course, be the case. But nobody can know at present. Clinical research in man has just begun, so time will tell whether or not the 'minors' can add to our current HLA-centered manipulations in transplantation immunology. Everybody seems to be convinced that there are more regulating systems behind tolerance induction than the HLA system. Perhaps the 'minors' are those which will come out of the black box in the end. We are eager to learn. If I understand correctly, however, 'minors' are only expressed in association with 'majors'. So even if Streilein is absolutely correct with his 'minors' hypothesis, that would not allow us to totally bypass the 'majors'.

A consequent exploitation of the HLA system by broad-based typing and matching will be inevitable to exploit all chances to improve tolerance induction in penetrating keratoplasty.

Rainer Sundmacher, MD, FRCOphth
Universität Düsseldorf, Klinik für Augenheilkunde,
Moorenstrassse 5, D–40225 Düsseldorf (Germany)
Tel. +49 211 811 7320, Fax +49 211 811 6421, E-Mail sundmach@uni-duesseldorf.de

Subject Index